Current Clinical Strategies

Outpatient and Primary Care Medicine

2001 Edition

Paul D. Chan, MD
David M. Thomas, MD
Eric W. McKinley, MD
Elizabeth K. Stanford, MD

D1446630

Current Clinical Strategies Publishing

www.ccspublishing.com

Digital Book and Updates

Purchasers of this book may download the digital book and updates of this text at the Current Clinical Strategies Publishing internet site: www.ccspublishing.com.

Current Clinical Strategies Publishing
27071 Cabot Road
Laguna Hills, California 92653-7012
Phone: 800-331-8227
Fax: 800-965-9420
Internet: www.ccspublishing.com
E-mail: info@ccspublishing.com

Printed in USA   ISBN 1-881528-89-8

Contents

Cardiovascular Disorders

Coronary Artery Disease

Coronary artery disease, either with or without angina, includes patients with prior myocardial infarction, prior revascularization, angiographically proven coronary atherosclerosis, or noninvasive evidence of myocardial ischemia. The patient may report previous chest pressure, heaviness, and/or pain, with or without radiation of the pain and/or shortness of breath.

I. **Clinical evaluation**
   A. History taking and physical examination, including medication are important to confirm the diagnosis, assist in risk stratification, and develop a treatment plan. Important points include the following:
      1. History of previous heart disease
      2. Possible non-atheromatous causes of angina (eg, aortic stenosis)
      3. Comorbid conditions affecting progression of CAD
      4. Symptoms of systemic atherosclerosis
      5. Severity and pattern of symptoms of angina
   B. **Physical examination** should include a cardiovascular examination as well as evaluation for evidence of hyperlipidemia, hypertension, peripheral vascular disease, congestive heart failure, anemia, and thyroid disease.
   C. **Laboratory studies** should include an electrocardiogram and a fasting lipid profile (total cholesterol, high-density lipoprotein, calculated low-density lipoprotein, and triglycerides). Further studies may include chest films, hemoglobin, and tests for diabetes, thyroid function, and renal function.
   D. **Modifiable risk factors**, for coronary heart disease and comorbid factors should be addressed. Risk factors for coronary heart disease include smoking, inappropriate activity level, stress, hyperlipidemia, obesity, hypertension, and diabetes mellitus. Comorbid conditions that could affect myocardial ischemia include hypertension, anemia, thyroid disease, and hypoxemia.

II. **Exercise electrocardiography**
   A. Sensitivity of exercise electrocardiography (Master "2-step" exercise test, graded exercise [treadmill] test) may be reduced for patients unable to reach the level of exercise required for near maximal effort, such as:
      1. Patients taking beta blockers
      2. Patients in whom fatigue, dyspnea, or claudication symptoms develop
      3. Patients with vascular, orthopedic, or neurologic conditions who cannot perform leg exercises
   B. Reduced specificity may be seen in patients with abnormalities on baseline electrocardiograms, such as those taking digitalis medications, and in patients with left ventricular hypertrophy or left bundle branch block.

III. **Noninvasive imaging.** A noninvasive imaging study such as myocardial perfusion scintigraphy or stress echocardiography may be indicated in patients unable to complete exercise electrocardiography. Exercise electrocardiography and prognostic imaging studies may yield results that indicate high, intermediate, or low risk of adverse clinical events. High-risk patients should have a cardiology consultation. Patients who are at intermediate risk may benefit from noninvasive imaging. Low-risk patients can be managed medically with a good prognosis.

IV. **Medical therapy**
   A. **One aspirin tablet daily** is strongly recommended unless there are medical contraindications. In patients with mild, stable CAD, drug therapy may be limited to short-acting sublingual nitrates on an as-needed basis or prophylactically in situations known to cause angina. Use of a lower dose (0.3 mg) may reduce the incidence of side effects, such as

headache or hypotension.

B. **A beta-blocker** is indicated in asymptomatic patients with recent myocardial infarction. The use of angiotensin-converting enzyme inhibitors has been demonstrated to be beneficial in patients with left ventricular systolic dysfunction, including that caused by myocardial infarction. Beta blockers are now recommended as first-line therapy or monotherapy for patients with stable CAD. Drugs without intrinsic sympathomimetic activity should be used. Cardioselective agents are a preferred in patients with diabetes or pulmonary disease.

1. **Non-cardioselective beta-blockers**
   a. **Propranolol sustained-release (Inderal LA)**, 60-160-mg qd [60, 80, 120, 160 mg].
   b. **Nadolol (Corgard)**, 40-80 mg qd [20, 40, 80, 120, 160 mg].
2. **Cardioselective beta-blockers**
   a. **Metoprolol (Lopressor)**, 100 mg bid [25, 50, 100 mg] or metoprolol XL (Toprol XL) 100-200 mg qd [50, 100, 200 mg tab ER].
   b. **Atenolol (Tenormin)**, 100 mg qd [25, 50, 100 mg].
   c. **Bisoprolol (Zebeta)** 5-20 mg qd [5, 10 mg].
3. **Adverse Effects**. Beta blockers are usually well tolerated. Symptomatic bradycardia, hypotension, fatigue, heart failure, dyspnea, cold extremities, and bronchospasm may occur. Impotence, constipation, and vivid dreams may occasionally occur.
4. **Contraindications to beta-blockers**
   a. Raynaud's phenomenon, reactive airway disease, or resting leg or foot pain caused by peripheral vascular disease.
   b. Beta blockers (including cardioselective agents) can cause severe bronchospasm in patients with reactive airway disease.

C. **Long-acting nitrates.** If beta blockers cannot be prescribed as first-line therapy, nitrates are the preferred alternative because of their efficacy. Sublingual nitroglycerin can be used prophylactically prior to activities that are likely to precipitate angina.

1. **Immediate-release nitroglycerin**
   a. Nitroglycerin, sublingually or in spray form, is the only agent that is effective for rapid relief of an established angina attack.
   b. Patients should carry nitroglycerin tablets or spray at all times and use it as needed.
   c. Nitroglycerin SL (Nitrostat), 0.3-1.5 mg SL q5min prn pain [0.15, 0.3, 0.4, 0.6 mg].
   d. Nitroglycerin oral spray (Nitrolingual) 1-2 sprays prn pain.
2. **Nitroglycerin patches:** Tolerance may be avoided by removing the patch at 2 p.m. for 8 hours each day. A minimum of 15 mg of nitroglycerin per 24-hr period is necessary for effect. Nitroglycerin patch (Transderm-Nitro) 0.6-0.8 mg/h applied for 16 hours each day [0.4, 0.6, 0.8 mg/h patches].
   a. **Isosorbide dinitrate**
      (1) Isosorbide dinitrate slow-release, (Dilatrate-SR, Isordil Tembids) one tab bid-tid.
      (2) Isosorbide dinitrate (Isordil, Titradose) 10-60 mg PO tid-qid [5, 10, 20, 30, 40 mg]; sustained release, 40-80 mg PO q8-12h [40 mg].
      (3) Isosorbide dinitrate immediate-release, 30 mg tid-qid.
   b. **Isosorbide mononitrate immediate release (ISMO, Monoket)**, 10 to 20 mg bid in the morning and again 7 hours later [10, 20 mg].
   c. **Isosorbide mononitrate extended-release (Imdur)**: Start with 30 mg, and increase the dose to 120 mg once daily [30, 60,120 mg].
   d. **Adverse effects.** Nitrates are well tolerated. The most common adverse effect is headache (30-60%). Symptomatic postural hypotension may sometimes occur. Syncope may rarely occur.

D. **Calcium channel blockers.** For patients who are unable to take beta blockers or long-acting nitrates, the use of long-acting calcium channel blockers has been shown to be clinically effective.
   1. Nifedipine XL (Procardia XL) 30-120 mg qd [30, 60, 90 mg].
   2. Diltiazem SR (Cardizem SR) 60-120 mg bid [60, 90, 120 mg].
   3. Diltiazem CD (Cardizem CD) 120-300 mg qd [120, 180, 240, 300 mg]
   4. Verapamil SR (Calan SR, Isoptin SR), 120-240 mg qd [120, 180, 240 mg].
   5. Diltiazem and verapamil are contraindicated in second degree or higher atrioventricular block. Calcium channel blockers should be used with caution in heart failure.
E. **Combination therapy** may be necessary in selected patients. A combination of beta blockers and long-acting nitrates is preferred because of efficacy and reduced potential for adverse side effects.
F. **Percutaneous transluminal coronary angiography and artery bypass grafting.** The relative survival benefit of CABG, compared with medical therapy, is enhanced by an increase in the absolute number of severely narrowed coronary arteries, the degree of left ventricular systolic dysfunction, and the magnitude of myocardial ischemia. No survival benefit has been documented with PTCA in stable CAD. PTCA is an alternative to medical therapy in patients with clinical evidence of ischemia and with angiographically suitable lesions.

References: See page 195.

Heart Failure

Heart failure (HF) has an incidence of 1% at age 50 and roughly doubles for each decade of life thereafter. The 5-year mortality rate is 62% in men and 42% in women.

I. **Pathophysiology of heart failure**
   A. HF is defined as insufficient cardiac function to supply the metabolic demands of the body. Systolic dysfunction produces ventricular dilation with poor contractile function.
   B. Impaired ventricular filling, or diastolic dysfunction, is common, especially in elderly hypertensive patients, and may be seen in 30% of patients who have clinical evidence of HF. It is characterized by ventricular hypertrophy, with preserved cardiac contractility. Impaired diastolic filling leads to a reduction in stroke volume and a corresponding reduction in cardiac output. Routine echocardiography is required in any patient with new-onset HF, since measurement of left ventricular function helps differentiate systolic from diastolic dysfunction.

II. **Clinical manifestations and evaluation**
   A. **Symptoms of heart failure** include weakness, fatigue, lethargy, light-headedness, mental confusion, and ultimately "cardiac cachexia"--generalized exhaustion with loss of muscle mass. The earliest subjective symptom attributable to pulmonary congestion is dyspnea caused by interstitial edema. As the condition progresses, orthopnea and paroxysmal nocturnal dyspnea (PND) may also develop.

New York Heart Association Criteria for Heart Failure	
Class I	Asymptomatic
Class II	Symptoms with moderate activity
Class III	Symptoms with minimal activity
Class IV	Symptoms at rest

B. **Common clinical signs** of HF include peripheral edema, pulmonary rales, an S3 gallop, sinus tachycardia, increased jugular venous pressure, and abdominojugular reflux. Signs of chronic HF are often found in noncardiac disorders such as obesity, venous insufficiency, and pulmonary disease.

C. **Other disorders may mimic HF** include volume overload from renal disease, regurgitant valvular disease, aortic stenosis, high output failure (anemia, sepsis, hyperthyroidism), pericardial disease, and tachyarrhythmias.

Laboratory Workup for Suspected HF	
Blood urea nitrogen	Magnesium
Cardiac enzymes (CK-MB, troponin, or both)	Thyroid-stimulating hormone
	Urinalysis
Complete blood cell count	Echocardiogram
Creatinine	Electrocardiography
Electrolytes	
Liver function tests	

III. Treatment of chronic heart failure

A. Nonpharmacologic treatments include salt restriction (a diet with 2 g sodium or less), alcohol restriction, water restriction for patients with severe renal impairment or psychogenic polydipsia, and regular aerobic exercise as tolerated.

B. **Diuretics**
1. Diuretics are the most rapidly effective drugs for treating the symptoms of pulmonary congestion. They are no longer recommended as initial therapy for chronic heart failure because the resulting volume depletion may increase sympathetic stimulation. For long-term therapy, diuretics should be combined with ACE inhibitors or angiotensin II receptor antagonists (ARAs).
2. Patients with moderate-to-severe HF will usually require furosemide, 20-160 mg, for adequate diuresis. The dosage may be increased and often doubled. In patients who respond poorly to high doses of furosemide, the addition of metolazone (Zaroxolyn) or HCTZ, 2.5-5.0 mg, 30-60 minutes before the morning dose of diuretic is often effective.
3. Torsemide (Demadex), 10-100 mg, is comparable to furosemide but with a longer duration of action.

C. **ACE inhibitors and angiotensin II receptor antagonists**
1. ACE inhibitors reduce preload, afterload, right atrial pressure, pulmonary capillary wedge pressure, arterial blood pressure, and systemic vascular resistance.

ACE Inhibitors		
Drug	Initial dose	Ususal dose (max dose)
Captopril (Capoten)	6.25 mg bid, tid	12.5-25 mg bid, tid (150 mg/d)
Enalapril (Vasotec)	2.5-5 mg qd	10-20 mg bid (40 mg/d)
Lisinopril (Prinivil/Zestril)	5-10 mg qd	20-40 mg qd (80 mg/d)
Ramipril (Altace)	1.25-2.5 mg bid	5 mg bid (20 mg/d)
Benazepril (Lotensin)	10 mg qd	20-40 mg qd, (40 mg/d) bid
Fosinopril (Monopril)	10 mg qd	20-40 mg qd (40 mg/d)
Quinapril (Accupril)	5 mg bid	20-40 mg bid (80 mg/d)
Perindopril (Aceon)	1 mg qd	1-4 mg qd (16 mg/d)
Moexipril (Univasc)	7.5 mg qd	7.5-15 mg qd (30 mg/d)
Trandolapril (Mavik)	1-2 mg qd (2 mg in backs)	2-4 mg qd (8 mg/d)

    2. In patients who cannot tolerate or have contraindications to ACE inhibitors, ARAs should be considered. ARAs offer advantages that appear similar to the ACE inhibitors. Side effects such as cough and angioedema are rare.

D. Digoxin
    1. Digoxin, 0.25 mg po daily, increases the force and velocity of myocardial contractions, although this positive inotropic effect is mild. Digoxin has very limited utility in the treatment of acute symptomatic HF. It is an agent of choice when tachyarrhythmia is associated with HF. Digoxin is contraindicated in patients with pure diastolic dysfunction, because the increased contractility is detrimental to cardiac function.
    2. Signs of toxicity include nausea, vomiting, anorexia, disturbances in color vision, weakness, fatigue, dizziness, new-onset psychosis, and cardiac arrhythmias.

E. Beta-blockers
    1. Long-term use of beta-blockers in patients with end-stage HF may improve LV function and increase survival. The mechanisms responsible for this beneficial effect may derive from opposition to the toxic effects of persistent catecholamine secretion.
    2. **Carvedilol (Coreg)** is the only beta-blocker that is FDA-approved for systolic dysfunction. Carvedilol reduces symptoms and improves LV function and also appears to improve survival.
    3. **Beta-blockers** should be reserved for patients who do not respond to more traditional agents. In addition, if a beta-blocker is used for HF with systolic dysfunction, it must be started at a low dose and titrated exceedingly slowly over a period of months. Symptoms may initially worsen before they improve. Beta-blockers are a treatment of choice for

HF from diastolic dysfunction. Beneficial effects include a slowed heart rate and increased cardiac output.

References: See page 195.

Hypertension

Hypertension is a major risk factor for coronary artery disease (CAD), heart failure, stroke, and renal failure. Approximately 50 million Americans have hypertension.

I. **Clinical evaluation of the hypertensive patient**
   A. Evaluation of hypertension should include an assessment of missed doses of maintenance antihypertensive therapy, use of nonsteroidal anti-inflammatory drugs, decongestants, diet medications, cocaine, or amphetamines.
   B. History should exclude the presence of coronary heart disease (chest pain), hyperlipidemia, diabetes, smoking, or prostatic hypertrophy. These disorders may influence the choice of antihypertensive.
   C. **Physical examination**. The diagnosis of hypertension requires three separate readings of at least 140/90. The physical exam should search for retinal hemorrhages, carotid bruits, left ventricular enlargement, coarctation of the aorta, aortic aneurysm, and absence of a peripheral pulse in an extremity.

Classification of Blood Pressure (mmHg) in the JNC VI				
Category	Systolic		Diastolic	Follow-up recommendation
Optimal	<120	and	<80	
Normal	<130	and	<85	Recheck in 2 y
High-normal	130-139	or	85-89	Recheck in 1 y
Hypertension				
Stage 1	140-159	or	90-99	Confirm within 2 mo
Stage 2	160-179	or	100-109	Evaluate within 1 mo
Stage 3	≥180	or	≥110	Evaluate immediately or within weeks
Isolated systolic hypertension	≥140	and	<90	Depends on stage

II. **Initial diagnostic evaluation of hypertension**
   A. **12 lead electrocardiography** may document evidence of ischemic heart disease, rhythm and conduction disturbances, or left ventricular hypertrophy.
   B. **Screening labs** include a complete blood count, glucose, potassium, calcium, creatinine, BUN, and a fasting lipid panel.
   C. **Urinalysis.** Dipstick testing should include glucose, protein, and hemoglo-

bin

    D. Selected patients may require plasma renin activity, 24 hour urine catecholamines, or renal function testing (glomerular filtration rate and blood flow).

III. Secondary hypertension

    A. Only 1-2% of all hypertensive patients will prove to have a secondary cause of hypertension. Age of onset greater than 60 years, age of onset less than 20 in African-American patients, or less than 30 in white patients suggests a secondary cause. Blood pressure that is does not respond to a three-drug regimen or a sudden acceleration of blood pressure suggests secondary hypertension.

    B. **Hypokalemia** (potassium <3.5 mEq/L while not taking diuretics) suggests primary aldosteronism. Cushingoid features suggests Cushing's disease. Spells of anxiety, sweating, or headache suggests pheochromocytoma.

    C. **Aortic coarctation** is suggested by a femoral pulse delayed later than the radial pulse, or by posterior systolic bruits below the ribs. Renovascular stenosis is suggested by paraumbilical abdominal bruits.

    D. **Pyelonephritis** is suggested by persistent urinary tract infections or costovertebral angle tenderness. Renal parenchymal disease is suggested by an increased serum creatinine ≥1.5 mg/dL and proteinuria.

Evaluation of Secondary Hypertension	
Renovascular Hypertension	Captopril Test: Plasma renin level before and 1 hr after captopril 25 mg. A greater than 150% increase in renin is positive Captopril Renography: Renal scan before and after 25 mg MRI angiography Arteriography (DSA)
Hyperaldosteronism	Serum potassium Serum aldosterone and plasma renin activity CT scan of adrenals
Pheochromocytoma	24 hr urine catecholamines CT scan Nuclear MIBG scan
Cushing's Syndrome	Plasma cortisol Dexamethasone suppression test
Hyperparathyroidism	Serum calcium Serum parathyroid hormone

IV. Non-pharmacologic treatment of hypertension

    A. Lifestyle modification

        1. The mean drop in blood pressure with lifestyle modification is 9 mm Hg. Weight loss, in the range of 10 pounds, can lead to a significant reduction in blood pressure. Exercise should consist of a minimum of 30 minutes of brisk walking, 3 times per week. Limitation of liquor to 2 oz a day has been shown to reduce blood pressure.

        2. Sodium intake should be limited to 2 gm per day by omitting high sodium foods, salt seasoning, and prepackaged fast-foods.

        3. Smoking cessation is recommended in patients who smoke.

V. Treatment recommendations of the Sixth National Committee on high blood pressure

1. The committee recommends a diuretic or beta-blocker as initial treatment for uncomplicated hypertension because these agents have been shown to decrease morbidity and mortality. In patients with certain comorbidities, however, angiotensin-converting-enzyme (ACE) inhibitors, calcium-channel blockers, or α_1-blockers can be used as first-line agents.

2. **Diuretics**

   a. Diuretics lower BP by inhibiting renal sodium and water reabsorption. Diuretics are considered first-line therapy in patients with uncomplicated hypertension or with systolic heart failure. They are drugs of choice for isolated systolic hypertension. Diuretics are effective agents in African-American and elderly patients, since they tend to be more renin-dependent than Caucasian hypertensive patients.

   b. Hydrochlorothiazide (HCTZ) effectively lowers BP at doses as low as 12.5-25.0 mg qd. Its BP-lowering effect tends to plateau at doses above 25 mg/d.

   c. Indapamide (Lozol) and metolazone (Zaroxolyn) are thiazide-like diuretics that are also dosed once a day but offer the advantage of being effective at a creatinine clearance as low as 20 mL/min.

Thiazide Diuretics		
Drug	Usual dose	Maximum dose
Chlorthalidone (Hygroton)	12.5-25 mg qd	50 mg/d
Chlorothiazide (Diuril)	0.5-1 g/d (qd or bid)	2 g/d
Hydrochlorothiazide (HCTZ, Hydrodiuril)	12.5-25 mg qd	50 mg/d
Indapamide (Lozol)	1.25 mg qd	5 mg/d
Methyclothiazide (Enduron)	2.5 mg qd	5 mg/d
Metolazone (Zaroxolyn)	2.5-5 mg qd	5 mg/d

   d. Thiazide diuretics may cause hypokalemia, hypomagnesemia, hyperuricemia, hypercalcemia, hyperlipidemia, and hyperglycemia. With long-term use, these side effects will usually return to baseline. Potassium or magnesium supplements may be necessary when a thiazide diuretic is used, but combining these agents with amiloride or triamterene may preclude the need for supplementation.

A. β-Adrenergic receptor blockers

1. β-blockers are recommended first-line agents in uncomplicated hypertension, or in hypertensive patients with angina pectoris, cardiac arrhythmias, mitral valve prolapse, a history of myocardial infarction (MI), diastolic dysfunction, or migraine headaches. β-blockers are preferred in young Caucasian hypertensive patients (younger than 40-50). African-Americans tend to respond less well to β-blockers.

2. Common adverse effects of β-blockers include decreased exercise tolerance, cold extremities, depression, sleep disturbance, and impotence, although these side effects may be less severe with the β_1-selective blockers (ie, metoprolol, atenolol, bisoprolol). The use of β_1-selective agents also helps minimize adverse effects associated with

β_2-blockade (suppression of insulin release, promotion of bronchospasm). All β-blockers can exacerbate asthma, peripheral vascular disease, and diabetes at high doses.
3. β-blockers should be used with caution in patients with bronchospastic disease, and nonselective agents are contraindicated in these patients. Agents with ISA (acebutolol, pindolol, carteolol, penbutolol) partially stimulate the β-receptor while they antagonize it. The advantages of these agents include less resting bradycardia as well as neutral effects on lipid and glucose metabolism.

β-blockers		
Drug	Usual dose	Maximum dose
Acebutolol (Sectral)	200-800 mg/d (qd or bid)	1.2 g/d (bid)
Atenolol (Tenormin)	50-100 mg qd	100 mg qd
Betaxolol (Kerlone)	10 mg qd	20 mg qd
Bisoprolol (Zebeta)	5 mg qd	20 mg qd
Carteolol (Cartrol)	2.5 mg qd	10 mg qd
Metoprolol succinate (Toprol XL)	100-200 mg qd	400 mg qd
Metoprolol tartrate (Lopressor)	100-200 mg/d (qd or bid)	450 mg/d (qd or bid)
Nadolol (Corgard)	40 mg qd	320 mg/d
Penbutolol sulfate (Levatol)	20 mg qd	NA
Pindolol (Visken)	5 mg bid	60 mg/d
Propranolol (Inderal, Inderal LA)	120-160 mg qd (LA 640 mg/d)	
Timolol (Blocadren)	10-20 mg bid	60 mg/d (bid)

B. ACE inhibitors
   1. ACE inhibitors act by decreasing angiotensin II production, which then leads to decreased sodium and water retention, decreased potassium excretion, and arterial vasodilation. In patients with systolic dysfunction, cardiac output actually improves with ACE inhibition.
   2. Monotherapy with ACE inhibitors is generally less effective in African-American hypertensive patients than in Caucasian hypertensives.
   3. ACE inhibitors are recommended for hypertensive patients with left ventricular dysfunction, previous MI, and diabetes. In type 1 diabetes, captopril (Capoten) and enalapril (Vasotec) have been shown to delay the progression to renal failure. In post-MI patients and those with systolic dysfunction and decreased ejection fraction (40% or less), ACE inhibitors significantly decrease mortality and reduce hospital admissions for heart failure and MI.
   4. **Adverse effects of ACE inhibitors**
      a. **Hypotension** is especially a problem with elderly patients, volume

depleted patients, and those on diuretics. These agents can worsen renal function. They should be used with caution in patients with serum creatinine levels of >3.0 mg/dL. ACE inhibitors should be used with caution in unilateral renal artery stenosis (RAS) and are contraindicated in bilateral RAS. Patients should be monitored for hyperkalemia.

b. **A dry, bothersome cough** is the most common adverse effect, occurring in 6-20%.

c. **Angioedema** is a rare (0.1%-0.2%) but potentially fatal side effect.

Angiotensin-Converting Enzyme Inhibitors		
Drug	Usual doses	Maximum dose
Benazepril (Lotensin)	20-40 mg qd or divided bid	80 mg/d
Captopril (Capoten)	50 mg bid-qid	450 mg/d
Enalapril (Vasotec, Vasotec IV)	10-40 mg qd or divided bid	40 mg/d
Fosinopril (Monopril)	20-40 mg qd or divided bid	80 mg/d
Lisinopril (Prinivil, Zestril)	20-40 mg qd	40 mg/d
Moexipril (Univasc)	15-30 mg qd	30 mg/d
Quinapril (Accupril)	20-80 mg qd or divided bid	80 mg/d
Ramipril (Altace)	5-20 mg qd or divided bid	20 mg/d
Trandolapril (Mavik)	2-4 mg qd	8 mg/d

VI. Angiotensin II receptor blockers

A. Angiotensin II receptor blockers (ARBs) decrease BP by inhibiting the coupling of AII to the angiotensin receptor. ARBs are as effective as other major classes of antihypertensives at reducing BP. In contrast to ACE inhibitors, ARBs have not been shown to slow the progression to renal failure in patients with diabetes. ARBs do not cause cough or angioedema, but they may cause hyperkalemia.

B. These agents are appropriate alternatives for patients who are candidates for an ACE inhibitor but cannot tolerate these agents due to cough or angioedema.

Angiotensin II Receptor Blockers		
Drug	Usual dose	Maximum dose
Candesartan (Atacand)	4-8 mg qd	16 mg/d
Irbesartan (Avapro)	150-300 mg qd	300 mg/d

Drug	Usual dose	Maximum dose
Losartan (Cozaar)	50 mg qd	100 mg/d
Valsartan (Diovan)	80 mg qd	320 mg/d

VII. **Calcium-channel blockers**
   A. Calcium-channel blockers (CCBs) can reduce myocardial contractility, produce vasodilation, and decrease systemic vascular resistance. When β-blockers cannot be used, CCBs are rational choices in hypertensive patients with concomitant angina. Due to their negative inotropic and chronotropic actions, diltiazem and verapamil are preferred in hypertensive patients who have diastolic dysfunction. Diltiazem and verapamil have been shown to reduce renal protein loss in patients with diabetes.
   B. **Peripheral edema** develops in up to 20% of patients. Headaches, dizziness, and flushing are also common adverse effects. Diltiazem and verapamil can worsen symptoms of heart failure. Short-acting preparations of CCBs should be avoided because they increase the risk of MI.

VIII. **Alpha-1-blockers**
   A. Alpha-1-blockers lower BP by inhibiting α_1-receptors on veins and arteries. Their mechanism of action is mainly due to peripheral vasodilation. Antagonism of these receptors results in relief of symptoms of benign prostatic hyperplasia (BPH).
   B. Alpha-1-blockers have been found as effective as other major classes of antihypertensives in lowering BP. Alpha$_1$-Blockers have a characteristic first-dose effect, which means that orthostatic hypotension frequently occurs with the first few doses of the drug. This side effect is minimized by slowly titrating the dose and by administering the first few doses at bedtime.

Alpha-1-blockers		
Drug	Initial dose	Maximum dose
Terazosin (Hytrin)	1 mg qhs; titrate slowly; Usual: 1-5 mg qhs	20 mg/d
Doxazosin (Cardura)	1 mg qd; titrate slowly every 2 weeks	16 mg/d

Combination Agents for Hypertension		
Drug	Initial dose	Comments
Beta-Blocker/Diuretic		
Atenolol/Chlorthalidone (Tenoretic)	50 mg/25 mg, 1 tab qd	Additive vasodilation
Bisoprolol/HCTZ (Ziac)	2.5 mg/6.25 mg, 1 tab qd	
Metoprolol/HCTZ (Lopressor HCTZ)	100 mg/25 mg, 1 tab qd	
Nadolol/HCTZ (Corzide)	40 mg/5 mg, 1 tab qd	

Drug	Initial dose	Comments
Propranolol/HCTZ (Inderide LA)	80 mg/50 mg, 1 tab qd	
Timolol/HCTZ (Timolide)	10 mg/25 mg, 1 tab qd	
ACE inhibitor/Diuretic		
Benazepril/HCTZ (Lotensin HCT)	5 mg/6.25 mg, 1 tab qd	ACE inhibitor conserves potassium and magnesium; combination beneficial for CHF patients with HTN; caution with elderly patients (orthostatic hypotension)
Captopril/HCTZ (Capozide)	25 mg/15 mg, 1 tab qd	
Enalapril/HCTZ (Vaseretic)	5 mg/12.5 mg, 1 tab qd	
Lisinopril/HCTZ (Zestoretic, Prinzide)	10 mg/12.5 mg, 1 tab qd	
Moexipril/HCTZ (Uniretic)	7.5 mg/12.5 mg, 1 tab qd	
ACE inhibitor/Calcium-channel blocker		
Benazepril/Amlodipine (Lotrel)	2.5 mg/10 mg, 1 tab qd	
Enalapril/Felodipine (Lexxel)	5 mg/5 mg, 1 tab qd	
Enalapril/Diltiazem (Teczem)	5 mg/180 mg, 1 tab qd	
Trandolapril/Verapamil (Tarka)	2 mg/180 mg, 1 tab qd	
Angiotensin II receptor blocker/Diuretic		
Losartan/HCTZ (Hyzaar)	50 mg/12.5 mg, 1 tab qd	
Valsartan/HCTZ (Diovan HCT)	80 mg/12.5 mg, 1 tab qd	
Alpha-1-Blocker/Diuretic		
Prazosin/Polythiazide (Minizide)	1 mg/0.5 mg, 1 cap bid	Synergistic vasodilation
K⁺-sparing diuretic/Thiazide		
Amiloride/HCTZ (Moduretic)	5 mg/50 mg, 1 tab qd	Electrolyte-sparing effect
Triamterene/HCTZ (Dyazide, Maxzide)	37.5 mg/25 mg, ½ tab qd	

Consideration of Concomitant Conditions in the Treatment of Hypertension	
Compelling indications	
Heart failure	ACE inhibitor, diuretic
Isolated systolic hypertension	Diuretic (first choice), long-acting calcium-channel blocker (second choice)
Post acute myocardial infarction	β-blocker (non-ISA); ACE inhibitor (in systolic dysfunction)
Type 1 diabetes mellitus	ACE inhibitor
Likely to be beneficial to patients with comorbidity	
Angina	β-blocker, calcium-channel blocker
Atrial fibrillation	β-blocker, calcium-channel blocker
Benign prostatic hyperplasia	α₁-blocker
Heart failure	Carvedilol, angiotensin II receptor blocker
Type 2 diabetes mellitus	ACE inhibitor (first choice); calcium-channel blocker

References: See page 195.

Atrial Fibrillation

Atrial fibrillation has a prevalence of 4 percent in the adult population. The prevalence of this arrhythmia increases with age, from less than 0.05 percent in patients 25 to 35 years of age to more than 5 percent in patients over 69 years of age. Atrial fibrillation is associated with an increased susceptibility to embolic stroke. The annual risk of stroke in patients with atrial fibrillation is 4.5 percent. Atrial fibrillation also can decrease exercise tolerance and has been associated with tachycardia-induced cardiomyopathy. Although many patients with atrial fibrillation are symptomatic, some patients remain asymptomatic.

I. Clinical evaluation
   A. Atrial fibrillation (AF) may manifest only as fatigue caused by impaired cardiac output or the patient may have no symptoms. Palpitations, shortness of breath or chest pain may occur, and syncope may infrequently accompany AF. Symptoms of myocardial ischemia and angina may be caused by the rapid ventricular rate. Paroxysmal AF may cause symptoms that abate and recur.
   B. The cause of the atrial fibrillation should be identified. Precipitating causes, such as hyperthyroidism, electrolyte abnormalities, and drug toxicity, should be excluded. Stimulant abuse, excess tobacco, alcohol, caffeine, chocolate, over-the-counter cold remedies, and street drugs should be sought. AF may be associated with a recent acute illness, such as pneumonia.

II. Physical examination
   A. The pulse is characterized by an irregular-irregular timing and amplitude. The rapid ventricular rate may cause hypotension and pulmonary congestion.

B. The patient should be examined for hypertension, valvular disease, pericarditis, coronary artery disease, hyperthyroidism, or chronic obstructive pulmonary disease. Murmurs and cardiac enlargement should be sought. Peripheral bruits may be a marker for associated coronary artery disease.

III. Diagnostic evaluation

A. 12-lead electrocardiogram reveals irregular R-R intervals with no P waves. The ventricular rate is irregularly, irregular and the ventricular response rate is usually 130-180 bpm.

B. Laboratory evaluation. Chest x-ray, electrolytes and screening labs, ECG, transesophageal echocardiogram, free T4, TSH, and drug levels (theophylline) should be assessed.

Causes of Atrial Fibrillation	
Hypoglycemia	Hypertrophic cardiomyopathy
Theophylline intoxication	Coronary artery disease
Acute pulmonary disease (pneumonia, asthma, chronic obstructive pulmonary disease, pulmonary embolus)	Atrial septal defect
	Aortic stenosis
Heavy alcohol intake or alcohol withdrawal	Infiltrative diseases (amyloidosis, cardiac tumors)
	Acute myocardial infarction
Hyperthyroidism	Lone atrial fibrillation (No underlying disease state)
Severe acute systemic illness	
Left or right ventricular failure	Electrolyte abnormalities
Mitral valve disease (stenosis or regurgitation)	Stimulant abuse, excess tobacco, xanthine (tea), chocolate, over-the-counter cold remedies, street drugs.
Pericarditis	
Hypertensive heart disease with left ventricular hypertrophy	

IV. Treatment of acute atrial fibrillation: rate and rhythm control

A. Patients who are unstable (ie, a heart rate of 150 or more with low blood pressure, angina pectoris, shortness of breath, decreased level of consciousness, shock, pulmonary congestion, congestive heart failure or acute myocardial infarction) during atrial fibrillation require immediate cardioversion using a 200-joule synchronized shock (with effective conscious sedation if time permits).

B. Restoration and maintenance of sinus rhythm often require the use of antiarrhythmic medications that carry a risk of proarrhythmia.

C. External direct current (DC) cardioversion is the most effective means of cardioverting atrial fibrillation to sinus rhythm. In patients with atrial fibrillation refractory to internal transvenous cardioversion, it is an alternative means of restoring sinus rhythm.

D. Prevention of embolic events during cardioversion

   1. Both electric and pharmacologic cardioversion carry a risk of embolic events, including stroke. Patients with persistent atrial fibrillation of unknown duration or more than 48 hours duration should be treated with anticoagulants for three weeks before either pharmacologic or DC cardioversion is attempted. Anticoagulation should be continued for four weeks after cardioversion. The International Standardized Ratio (INR) should be maintained between 2.0 and 3.0.

   2. Transesophageal echocardiography may be used to exclude the presence of thrombus in the atria of patients being considered for cardioversion. A negative transesophageal echocardiogram does not obviate the need for at least a short course of warfarin (Coumadin) therapy after cardioversion.

V. Pharmacologic methods of ventricular rate control

A. The first goals of therapy should be control of the ventricular rate. Intravenous calcium channel blockers and beta blockers have the advantage of rapid onset of action. Digoxin has a delayed onset of action of two hours. Digoxin is not effective in converting atrial fibrillation to sinus rhythm. Therefore, digoxin is not recommended for the acute conversion of atrial fibrillation and should only be used in patients with decreased left ventricular function.

Agents Used for Heart Rate Control in Atrial Fibrillation

Agent	Loading Dose	Onset of Action	Maintenance Dosage	Major Side Effects
Diltiazem (Cardizem)	0.25 mg per kg IV over 2 minutes	2 to 7 minutes	10 to 15 mg per hour IV or 120 to 360 mg PO every day in divided doses	Hypotension, heart block, heart failure
Verapamil (Calan, Isoptin)	0.075 to 0.15 mg per kg IV over 2 minutes	3 to 5 minutes	240 to 360 mg PO every day in divided doses	Hypotension, heart block, heart failure
Esmolol (Brevibloc)	0.5 mg per kg IV over one minute	5 minutes	0.05 to 0.2 mg/kg/minute IV	Hypotension, heart block, bradycardia, asthma, heart failure
Metoprolol (Lopressor)	2.5 to 5 mg IV bolus over 2 minutes, up to 3 doses	5 minutes	50 to 200 mg PO every day in divided doses	Hypotension, heart block, bradycardia, asthma, heart failure
Propranolol (Inderal)	0.15 mg per kg	5 minutes	40 to 320 mg PO every day in divided doses	Hypotension, heart block, bradycardia, asthma, heart failure
Digoxin (Lanoxin)	0.25 mg IV or PO every 2 hours, up to 1.5 mg	5 to 30 minutes for IV therapy or 30 minutes to 2 hours	0.125 to 0.25 mg every day (oral or IV) for oral therapy	Digitalis toxicity, heart block, bradycardia

B. Pharmacologic Methods of Acute Cardioversion
   1. Pharmacologic agents may be used for acute cardioversion in patients with atrial fibrillation. All methods of pharmacologic cardioversion are associated with proarrhythmic risks.
C. Type IA medications
   1. **Intravenous procainamide** (Procainamide injection) is effective for cardioversion in up to 60%. In one hour, the conversion rate to sinus rhythm is only 20%. Side effects include hypotension and QRS and QT prolongation in patients with torsades de pointes.
   2. **Quinidine (Quinaglute).** The conversion rate with oral quinidine is up to 60%. Torsades de pointes is a major side effect.
D. Class IC Medications
   1. **Flecainide (Tambocor).** A single high-bolus dose of oral flecainide (less than 400 mg within three hours) has a conversion rate of 60 to 70

percent at three hours after treatment and up to 91 percent at eight hours.
2. **Propafenone (Rythmol)**. High-dose (600 mg) oral propafenone has a conversion rate of up to 76%.

Comparison of Antiarrhythmic Therapies

Class of agent	Agent	Dosage	Acute conversion rate	Chronic efficacy
IA	Procainamide (Procainamide injection)	10 to 15 mg per kg IV, at 25 mg per minute	20%	50%
	Quinidine (Quinaglute)	324 to 648 mg PO every 8 hours	38 to 86%	47 to 60%
IC	Propafenone (Rythmol)	600 mg PO as a single bolus dose; 150 to 300 mg three times daily as a maintenance dose	51 to 76%	50 to 60%
	Flecainide (Tambocor)	300 to 400 mg PO as a single bolus dose; 50 to 150 mg twice daily as a maintenance dose	68 to 91%	40 to 74%
III	Amiodarone (Cordarone)	150 mg IV over 10 minutes, then 30 to 60 mg IV per hour; 200 to 400 mg PO every day as a maintenance dose after loading	43 to 68%	55 to 65%
	Sotalol (Betapace)	160 to 320 mg PO daily in two doses	20 to 52%	50 to 60%
	Ibutilide (Corvert)	0.01 mg per kg IV for patients under 60 kg (132 lb), 1 mg for patients over 60 kg, over 10 minutes	33 to 45%	N/A
Other treatment	DC cardioversion	100 to 360 joules	67 to 94%	N/A

E. **Class III medications**
1. **Amiodarone (Cordarone)** does not appear to be effective in converting recent-onset atrial fibrillation to sinus rhythm. Oral amiodarone may be effective as an adjunct to DC cardioversion.
2. **Sotalol (Betapace)** is not useful for the acute termination of atrial fibrillation. Sotalol and amiodarone slow conduction and prolong refractoriness in the atrioventricular node and thus can control ventricular response to atrial fibrillation.
3. **Ibutilide (Corvert)** is an intravenous class III antiarrhythmic agent. It is indicated for the acute termination of atrial fibrillation and flutter. The half-life of ibutilide is three to six hours. Its clinical effect is gone in two

to six hours. Ibutilide is administered in a dosage of 0.01 mg per kg intravenously over 10 minutes. Conversion rates are between 33-45%. If the first dose is ineffective, a second may be administered before alternative strategies are considered.
   F. In summary, class IA and class IC agents are effective for acute termination of atrial fibrillation, with conversion rates of 60-80%. Although class III agents are useful as adjuncts to electric cardioversion and are effective in maintaining sinus rhythm, only ibutilide is useful for acute cardioversion.

References: See page 195.

Dyslipidemia

Dyslipidemias may be manifested by elevation of the serum total cholesterol, low-density lipoprotein (LDL) cholesterol and triglycerides, and a decrease in the high-density lipoprotein (HDL) cholesterol. Elevated serum cholesterol levels are associated with the development of coronary heart disease, and aggressive cholesterol reduction results in increased rates of plaque regression.
I. **Diagnosis and classification**
   A. Secondary causes of dyslipidemia include hypothyroidism and a genetic predisposition, such as autosomal dominant familial hypercholesterolemia. Triglyceride elevation may occur in association with diabetes mellitus, alcoholism, obesity and hypothyroidism.
   B. The National Cholesterol Education Program (NCEP) guidelines are based on clinical cut points that indicate relative risk for coronary heart disease. Total cholesterol and HDL cholesterol levels be measured every five years beginning at age 20 in patients who do not have coronary heart disease or other atherosclerotic disease. Both of these measurements may be obtained in the nonfasting state. The results of these measurements and the presence of other risk factors for coronary heart disease may demand a lipoprotein analysis.

Coronary Heart Disease Risk Based on Risk Factors Other Than the LDL Level

Positive risk factors
   Male ≥45 years
   Female ≥55 years or postmenopausal without estrogen replacement therapy
   Family history of premature coronary heart disease (definite myocardial infarction or sudden death before age 55 in father or other male first-degree relative or before age 65 in mother or other female first-degree relative)
   Current cigarette smoking
   Hypertension (blood pressure ≥140/90 mm Hg or patient is receiving antihypertensive drug therapy)
   HDL cholesterol level <35 mg/dL (<0.90 mmol/L)
   Diabetes mellitus
Negative risk factor*
   High HDL cholesterol level (≥60 mg/dL [≥1.60 mmol/L])

*--Subtract one positive risk factor if negative risk factor is present.
The LDL cholesterol level can be calculated by using the Friedwald formula (mg/dL): LDL=total cholesterol - HDL - (triglyceride/5)

II. **Management**
   A. The target LDL cholesterol value in patients with coronary heart disease or other atherosclerotic disease is 100 mg/dL or lower. If the LDL level does

not exceed 100 mg/dL in a patient with coronary heart disease, the patient should begin the step I diet, regularly participate in physical activity and stop smoking. Annual lipoprotein analysis is indicated for this group. Premenopausal women and men 35 years of age or younger with dyslipidemia but without other risk factors for coronary heart disease or a genetic predisposition are considered at low risk.

   B. The NCEP guidelines recommend that patients at higher risk of coronary heart disease receive more intensive interventions for dyslipidemia than patients at lower risk. Persons at highest risk for future coronary events have a history of coronary heart disease or extracoronary atherosclerotic disease.

Risk Classification of Hypercholesterolemia in Patients Without Coronary Heart Disease

Classifica-tion	Total choles-terol level	LDL choles-terol level	HDL choles-terol level
Desirable	200 mg/dL	<130 mg/dL	≥60 mg/dL
Borderline high risk	200 to 239 mg/dL	130 to 159 mg/dL	35 to 59 mg/dL
High risk	≥240 mg/dL	≥160 mg/dL	<35 mg/dL

III. Lifestyle modifications

   A. The NCEP guidelines recommend dietary modification, exercise and weight control as the foundation of treatment of dyslipidemia. These interventions may provide sufficient treatment for up to 90 percent of persons with dyslipidemia.

   B. **Exercise and weight reduction** lowers total cholesterol and its LDL and VLDL fractions, lowers triglycerides and raises HDL cholesterol. Most patients benefit from aerobic exercise that targets large muscle groups, performed for 30 minutes four or more times a week.

   C. **Step I and step II diets**
      1. Dietary therapy should be initiated in patients who have borderline-high LDL cholesterol levels (130 to 159 mg/dL) and two or more risk factors for coronary heart disease and in patients who have LDL levels of 160 mg/dL or greater. The objective of dietary therapy in primary prevention is to decrease the LDL cholesterol level to 160 mg/dL if only one risk factor for coronary heart disease is present and to less than 130 mg/dL if two or more risk factors are identified. In the presence of documented coronary heart disease, dietary therapy is indicated in patients who have LDL values exceeding 100 mg/dL, with the aim of lowering the LDL level to 100 mg/dL or less.
      2. **Step I diet** limits calories derived from saturated fats to 8 to 10 percent of total calories and cholesterol to less than 300 mg/day.
      3. **Step II diet** further restricts calories from saturated fats to less than 7 percent of total calories and restricts cholesterol intake to less than 200 mg/day.
      4. In primary prevention of coronary heart disease (without evidence of coronary heart disease), dietary therapy should be maintained for six months before drug therapy is initiated. In patients with coronary heart disease and an LDL cholesterol value above 100 mg/dL, therapy should begin with the step II diet.

IV. Drug therapy

A. Because dietary modification rarely reduces LDL cholesterol levels by more than 10 to 20 percent, the NCEP guidelines recommend that consideration be given to the use of cholesterol-lowering agents if lipid levels remain elevated after six months of intensive dietary therapy.

B. **A patient with a very high LDL cholesterol level** may need to start drug therapy sooner, because it is unlikely that a patient with an LDL level of 130 mg/dL or greater will be able to achieve the goal of 100 mg/dL with diet alone.

C. **HMG-CoA reductase inhibitors** are the drugs of choice in most patients with hypercholesterolemia because they reduce LDL cholesterol most effectively. Gemfibrozil (Lopid) or nicotinic acid may be better choices in patients with significant hypertriglyceridemia.

Cholesterol-Lowering Agents, Their Dosages and Cost	
Agent	**Maintenance dosage**
Bile acidbinding resins Cholestyramine (Questran, Questran Lite) Colestipol (Colestid)	4 g, 8 g , 12 g or 16 g twice daily 5 g twice daily or 30 g/day, in divided doses
HMG-CoA reductase inhibitors (statins) Atorvastatin (Lipitor) Cerivastatin (Baycol) Fluvastatin (Lescol) Lovastatin (Mevacor) Pravastatin (Pravachol) Simvastatin (Zocor)	10 to 80 mg/day anytime 0.3 mg in the evening 20 mg or 40 mg at bedtime, or 20 mg twice daily 20 mg, 40 mg or 80 mg with evening meal 10 mg, 20 mg or 40 mg at bedtime 5 mg, 10 mg, 20 mg or 40 mg at bedtime
Fibric acid analogs Clofibrate (Atromid-5) Gemfibrozil (Lopid)	500 mg four times daily 600 mg twice daily
Nicotinic acid	1.5 to 6 g daily in divided doses

Changes in Serum Lipid Values with Different Classes of Cholesterol-Lowering Drugs and Some of Their Side Effects					
Drug class	**Total cholesterol levels**	**LDL levels**	**HDL levels**	**Triglycerides**	**Side effects**
Bile acid binding resins	↓ 20%	↓ 10% to 20%	↑ 3% to 5%	Neutral or ↑	Unpalatability, bloating, constipation, heartburn
Nicotinic acid	↓ 25%	↓ 10% to 25%	↑ 15% to 35%	↓20% to 50%	Flushing, nausea, glucose intolerance, abnormal liver function test

Drug class	Total cholesterol levels	LDL levels	HDL levels	Triglycerides	Side effects
Fibric acid analogs	↓ 15%	↓ 5% to 15%	↑ 14% to 20%	↓ 20% to 50%	Nausea, skin rash
HMG-CoA reductase inhibitors	↓ 15% to 30%	↓ 20% to 60%	↑ 5% to 15%	↓ 10% to 40%	Myositis, myalgia, elevated hepatic transaminases

D. HMG-CoA reductase inhibitors

1. Lovastatin (Mevacor), pravastatin (Pravachol), simvastatin (Zocor), fluvastatin (Lescol), atorvastatin (Lipitor) and cerivastatin (Baycol) are HMG-CoA reductase inhibitors, or statins, that inhibit cholesterol synthesis. These agents lower total, LDL and triglyceride cholesterol and slightly raise the HDL fraction. While these agents are generally well tolerated, 1% may develop elevated hepatic transaminase levels, which may necessitate discontinuation of the drug. Other adverse effects include myopathy (0.1%) and gastrointestinal complaints.

2. Atorvastatin (Lipitor) may exert a greater effect on lowering LDL cholesterol, total cholesterol and triglycerides. Statins should generally be taken in a single dose with the evening meal or at bedtime.

E. Bile acidbinding resins

1. The anion exchange resins cholestyramine (Questran) and colestipol (Colestid) bind cholesterol-containing bile acids in the intestines. These agents decrease LDL cholesterol levels by up to 20 percent. They may be a good choice in patients with hepatic disease because they do not affect hepatic metabolism. They are also a good choice in very young patients and women of childbearing age.

2. Bile acidbinding resins may cause an increase in triglyceride levels. Side effects include constipation, abdominal discomfort, flatulence, nausea, bloating and heartburn.

3. Bile acid sequestrants can bind with warfarin, digitalis, thyroxine, thiazides, furosemide, tetracycline, penicillin G, phenobarbital, iron, propranolol, acetaminophen, nonsteroidal anti-inflammatory agents, oral phosphate, and hydrocortisone.

F. Nicotinic acid

1. Nicotinic acid, or niacin, decreases the synthesis of LDL cholesterol. This agent increases the HDL level by 15 to 35 percent, reduces total and LDL cholesterol levels by 10 to 25 percent, and decreases the triglyceride level by 20 to 50 percent.

2. Side effects of nicotinic acid include flushing, pruritus, gastrointestinal discomfort, hyperuricemia, gout, elevated liver function tests and glucose intolerance. Taking 325 mg of aspirin 30 minutes before the drug is ingested may minimize flushing. Therapy should be avoided in diabetes mellitus because it tends to worsen glycemic control.

G. Fibric acid derivatives

1. Fibric acid derivatives, or fibrates, increase the clearance of VLDL cholesterol by enhancing lipolysis and reducing hepatic cholesterol synthesis. These agents lower triglyceride levels by 20 to 50 percent,

raise HDL levels by up to 20 percent, and reduce LDL levels by approximately 5 to 15 percent. Gemfibrozil (Lopid) is particularly useful in patients with diabetes and familial dysbetalipoproteinemia.

2. Side effects of gemfibrozil include nausea, bloating, flatulence, abdominal distress and mild liver-function abnormalities. Myositis, gallstones and elevation of the LDL cholesterol level have also been reported. Fibrates should generally not be used with HMG-CoA reductase inhibitors because the risk of severe myopathy.

H. **Multiple drug therapy.** The NCEP guidelines define a target LDL cholesterol level of 100 mg/dL as a goal for high-risk patients with established coronary heart disease.

Combination Therapies If Single-Agent Therapy Is Not Effective in Reducing Lipid Levels	
Lipid levels	**First drug → drug to add**
Elevated LDL level and triglyceride level <200 mg/dL	Statin → bile acid binding resin Nicotinic acid* → statin* Bile acid binding resin → nicotinic acid
Elevated LDL level and triglyceride level 200 to 400 mg/dL	Statin* → nicotinic acid* Statin* → gemfibrozil (Lopid)††
LDL=low-density lipoprotein. *--Possible increased risk of myopathy and hepatitis. ††--Increased risk of severe myopathy.	

I. **Estrogen replacement therapy**. The NCEP recommends that consideration be given to estrogen replacement therapy as a means of decreasing (by about 15 percent) LDL cholesterol levels and increasing HDL cholesterol levels in postmenopausal women.

References: See page 195.

Pulmonary Disorders

Allergic Rhinitis and Conjunctivitis

Allergic rhinitis and allergic conjunctivitis are characterized by inflammation of the nasal mucosa, rhinorrhea, nasal congestion, sneezing, and conjunctival injection. The disorder is episodic, seasonal or perennial. Inhaled, ingested or injected allergens encounter IgE that is bound to mast cell membranes, resulting in mast cell degranulation, precipitating sneezing, itching, rhinorrhea and congestion.

I. **Diagnosis**
  A. Allergic rhinitis presents with nasal congestion, rhinorrhea, sneezing, nasal or ocular pruritus, excessive lacrimation, and postnasal drip with resulting sore throat and cough. Patients may also have asthma or atopic dermatitis in their personal or family history.
  B. **Physical examination**
    1. The conjunctivae may be injected, and profuse tearing may be present. Some patients present with swollen eyelids and boggy sclera. The nasal mucosa may be congested with a profuse clear discharge.
    2. Patients may exhibit "allergic shiners" (darkened circles under the eyes secondary to venous pooling) and a crease across the bridge of the nose caused by the "allergic salute" (chronic upward rubbing of the nose).
  C. **Laboratory testing**
    1. **Nasal smear.** Infectious rhinitis demonstrates a predominance of neutrophils, and allergic disease shows a predominance of eosinophils.
    2. **Allergy testing** is useful to identify patients with allergic disease that does not display a clear seasonal pattern. In patients with perennial symptoms, testing may help confirm allergic disease and allow identification of allergens that are potentially avoidable.

II. **Treatment**

Second-Generation Antihistamines	
Drug	**Adult dose**
Cetirizine (Zyrtec)	10 mg once daily
Fexofenadine (Allegra)	60 mg twice daily
Loratadine (Claritin)	10 mg once daily
Astemizole (Hismanal)	10 mg once daily

  A. Serious cardiac side effects have been reported with use of astemizole (Hismanal). Caution must be taken when coadministering astemizole with macrolides, antifungals, antidepressants or cimetidine because they may interfere with its metabolism.
  B. **Azelastine nasal spray (Astelin)** is an intranasal, topical antihistamine, which may cause somnolence; 2 sprays in each nostril bid.
  C. **Intranasal steroids** may be useful in relieving itching, rhinorrhea and congestion--and are more effective than antihistamines. Intranasal steroids require five to seven days for symptom improvement. The most common side effects are headache and local irritation. Occasionally, patients develop intranasal candidiasis.
  D. **Ophthalmic therapy**
    1. **Antihistamine-vasoconstrictor preparations.** Vasocon-A (naphazoline/antazoline) and Naphcon-A (naphazoline/pheniramine) are the most

commonly prescribed antihistamine-decongestants. These agents are available over the counter. 1-2 drops q2h as needed; up to 4 times a day. Rebound congestion can occur with long-term use.
   2. **Cromolyn (Crolom)**, a mast cell stabilizer, is highly effective for the treatment of allergic conjunctivitis; 1-2 drops in each eye q4-6h.
   3. **Lodoxamide (Alomide)**, a mast cell stabilizer, is more potent than cromolyn; 1-2 drops qid.
   4. **Levocabastine (Livostin)** is a histamine H1 antagonist. It provides relief within a few minutes.
   5. **Ketorolac (Acular)** is a topical NSAID; 1 drop qid is effective for seasonal allergic conjunctivitis.
E. **Topical ocular corticosteroids**
   1. Corticosteroids are very effective in treating ocular allergy. Dexamethasone (Decadron) 0.1% ophthalmic soln, 1-2 drops q4-8h.
   2. Because these drugs may elevate intraocular pressure and worsen infections, they should be administered with caution.

Intranasal Corticosteroids		
Drug	**Trade name**	**Dose (sprays/nostril)**
Beclomethasone	Beconase Vancenase Beconase AQ Vancenase AQ	One spray two to qid One spray bid-qid One to two sprays bid One to two sprays bid
Budesonide	Rhinocort	Two to four sprays bid
Flunisolide	Nasalide	Two sprays bid
Fluticasone	Flonase	Two sprays/day or one spray bid
Triamcinolone	Nasacort	Two to four sprays qd
Mometasone	Nasonex	Two sprays qd

III. **Immunotherapy.** Allergen immunotherapy is effective in patients with allergic rhinitis. Allergy treatment begins with identification of allergens, institution of avoidance procedures and administration of medication. Immunotherapy may be considered if other measures fail.

References: See page 195.

Acute Bronchitis

Acute bronchitis is one of the most common diagnoses made by primary care physicians. Viruses are the most common cause of acute bronchitis in otherwise healthy adults. Only a small portion of acute bronchitis infections are caused by nonviral agents, with the most common organisms being *Mycoplasma pneumoniae* and *Chlamydia pneumoniae*.

I. Diagnosis

A. The cough in acute bronchitis may produce either clear or purulent sputum This cough generally lasts seven to 10 days. Approximately 50 percent of patients with acute bronchitis have a cough that lasts up to three weeks, and 25 percent of patients have a cough that persists for over a month.

B. Physical examination. Wheezing, rhonchi, a prolonged expiratory phase or other obstructive signs may be present.

C. Diagnostic studies

   1. The appearance of sputum is not predictive of whether a bacterial infection is present. Purulent sputum is most often caused by viral infections. Microscopic examination or culture of sputum generally is not helpful. Since most cases of acute bronchitis are caused by viruses, cultures are usually negative or exhibit normal respiratory flora. When M. pneumoniae or C. pneumoniae infection is present, routine sputum cultures are still negative.

   2. Acute bronchitis can cause transient pulmonary function abnormalities which resemble asthma. Therefore, to diagnose asthma, changes that persist after the acute phase of the illness must be documented. When pneumonia is suspected, chest radiographs and pulse oximetry may be helpful.

II. Differential diagnosis

A. Acute bronchitis or pneumonia can present with fever, constitutional symptoms and a productive cough. Patients with pneumonia often have rales. When pneumonia is suspected on the basis of the presence of a high fever, constitutional symptoms or severe dyspnea, a chest radiograph should be obtained.

Differential Diagnosis of Acute Bronchitis	
Disease process	**Signs and symptoms**
Asthma	Evidence of reversible airway obstruction even when not infected
Allergic aspergillosis	Transient pulmonary infiltrates Eosinophilia in sputum and peripheral blood smear
Occupational exposures	Symptoms worse during the work week but tend to improve during weekends, holidays and vacations
Chronic bronchitis	Chronic cough with sputum production on a daily basis for a minimum of three months Typically occurs in smokers
Sinusitis	Tenderness over the sinuses, postnasal drainage
Common cold	Upper airway inflammation and no evidence of bronchial wheezing
Pneumonia	Evidence of infiltrate on the chest radiograph
Congestive heart failure	Basilar rales Orthopnea Cardiomegaly Evidence of increased interstitial or alveolar fluid on the chest radiograph S_3 gallop Tachycardia
Reflux esophagitis	Intermittent symptoms worse when lying down Heartburn

Disease process	Signs and symptoms
Bronchogenic tumor	Constitutional signs often present Cough chronic, sometimes with hemoptysis
Aspiration syndromes	Usually related to a precipitating event, such as smoke inhalation Vomiting Decreased level of consciousness

    B. Asthma should be considered in patients with repetitive episodes of acute bronchitis. Patients who repeatedly present with cough and wheezing can be given spirometric testing with bronchodilation to help differentiate asthma from recurrent bronchitis.

    C. Congestive heart failure may cause cough, shortness of breath and wheezing in older patients. Reflux esophagitis with chronic aspiration can cause bronchial inflammation with cough and wheezing. Bronchogenic tumors may produce a cough and obstructive symptoms.

III. Treatment

    A. Antibiotics. Physicians often treated acute bronchitis with antibiotics, even though scant evidence exists that antibiotics offer any significant advantage over placebo. Antibiotic therapy is beneficial in patients with exacerbations of chronic bronchitis.

Oral Antibiotic Regimens for Bronchitis	
Drug	**Recommended regimen**
Azithromycin (Zithromax)	Day 1,500 mg; then 250 mg qd
Erythromycin	250-500 mg q6h
Clarithromycin (Biaxin)	500 mg bid
Levofloxacin (Levaquin)	500 mg qd
Sparfloxacin (Zagam)	Day 1,400 mg; then 200 mg qd
Trovafloxacin (Trovan)	200 mg qd
Grepafloxacin (Raxar)	600 mg qd
Trimethoprim/sulfamethoxazole (Bactrim, Septra)	1 DS tablet bid
Doxycycline	100 mg bid

    B. Bronchodilators. Significant relief of symptoms occurs with inhaled albuterol (two puffs four times daily). Patients who are treated with inhaled albuterol also return to work sooner. When productive cough and wheezing are present, bronchodilator therapy may be useful.

References: See page 195.

Asthma

Asthma is the most common chronic disease among children. At least 75 percent of asthmatic patients demonstrate immediate hypersensitivity to common aeroallergens. Asthma triggers include viral infections; environmental pollutants, such as tobacco smoke; certain medications, (aspirin, nonsteroidal anti-inflammatory drugs), and sustained exercise, particularly in cold environments.

I. Diagnosis
  A. History
    1. Symptoms of episodic complaints of breathing difficulties, seasonal or nighttime cough, prolonged shortness of breath after a respiratory infection, or difficulty sustaining exercise.
    2. Reversible airways disease does not always represent asthma. Wheezing may persist for weeks after an acute bronchitis episode. Patients with chronic obstructive pulmonary disease may have a reversible component superimposed on their fixed obstruction. Etiologic clues include a personal history of allergic disease, such as rhinitis or atopic dermatitis, and a family history of allergic disease.
    3. The frequency of daytime and nighttime symptoms, duration of exacerbations and asthma triggers should be assessed.

Asthma Triggers

Sources of inhaled allergens	Environmental irritants/precipitants
House dust mites	Tobacco smoke
Animal danders from house pets	Cold air
Pollen	Exercise
Fungal spores	Particulates from wood stoves
Cockroaches	Air pollution
Animal urine from laboratory animals	Chemical gases or fumes
Infections	**Drugs**
Viral respiratory infections	Aspirin
Sinusitis	Nonsteroidal anti-inflammatory drugs
Gastroesophageal reflux	Angiotensin converting enzyme inhibitors
Sulfites (used as preservatives in food, beer and wine)	Beta blockers

  B. Physical examination. Hyperventilation, use of accessory muscles of respiration, audible wheezing, and a prolonged expiratory phase are common. Increased nasal secretions or congestion, polyps, and eczema may be present. The chest and lungs should be assessed for wheezing.
  C. Measurement of lung function. An increase in the forced expiratory volume in one second (FEV_1) of 12 percent after treatment with an inhaled beta$_2$ agonist is sufficient to make the diagnosis of reversible airways disease. A similar change in peak expiratory flow rate (PEFR) measured on a peak flow meter is also diagnostic.

Asthma Classification			
Symptoms			
Classifica-tion	Daytime	Nighttime	Lung function
Mild inter-mittent	Symptoms occur up to 2 times/week; exacerbations are brief (hours to days), with normal PEFR and no symptoms between exacerbations	Symptoms occur up to 2 times/month	PEFR or FEV$_1$ ≥80% of predicted; <20% variability in PEFR
Mild persis-tent	Symptoms occur more than 2 times/week but less than one time/day; exacerbations may affect normal activity	Symptoms occur more than 2 times/month	PEFR or FEV, ≥80% of predicted; PEFR variability 20-30%
Moderate persistent	Symptoms occur daily; daily need for inhaled short-acting beta$_2$ agonist; exacerbations affect normal activity; exacerbations occur more than 2 times/week and may last for days	Symptoms occur more than one time/week	PEFR or FEV$_1$ >60 but <80% of predicted; PEFR variability >30%
Severe per-sistent	Symptoms are continual; physical activity is limited; exacerbations are frequent	Symptoms are frequent	PEFR or FEV$_1$ <60% of predicted; PEFR variability >30%

II. Treatment
   A. **Allergen avoidance.** Patients should avoid opening windows and using unfiltered window fans. Elimination of allergens from house dust mites and cats also will reduce symptoms.
   B. **Long-term control medications**
      1. **Corticosteroids**
         a. Glucocorticoids provide anti-inflammatory effects and reduce bronchial hyperactivity. Inhaled corticosteroids are first-line agents in patients who require daily asthma therapy. No specific inhaled corticosteroid preparation is superior to another. Primary adverse effects of these medications are cough, oral thrush and hoarseness. In high doses, a potential exists for significant systemic absorption. Patients with severe persistent asthma may require daily systemic steroid therapy when other medications have failed.
         b. **Prednisone, prednisolone or methylprednisolone** (Solu-Medrol), 40 to 60 mg qd; for children, 1 to 2 mg/kg/day to a maximum of 60 mg/day. Therapy is continued for 3-10 days. The oral steroid dosage does not have to be tapered after short-course "burst" therapy if the patient is receiving inhaled steroid therapy.

Pharmacotherapy for Asthma Based on Disease Classification

Classification	Long-term control medications	Quick-relief medications
Mild intermittent		Short-acting beta$_2$ agonist as needed
Mild persistent	Low-dose inhaled corticosteroid or cromolyn sodium (Intal) or nedocromil (Tilade); alternatively, a leukotriene modifier may be used	Short-acting beta$_2$ agonist as needed
Moderate persistent	Medium-dose inhaled corticosteroid plus a long-acting bronchodilator (long-acting beta$_2$ agonist) if needed	Short-acting beta$_2$ agonist as needed
Severe persistent	High-dose inhaled corticosteroid plus a long-acting bronchodilator and systemic corticosteroid if needed	Short-acting beta$_2$ agonist as needed

Inhaled Corticosteroids and Mast Cell Stabilizers

Drug	Trade name	Dose (μg/puff)	Dose range (total puffs/day)		
			Low	Intermediate	High
Beclomethasone	Beclovent	42	4 to 12	12 to 20	>20
	Vanceril	42	4 to 12	12 to 20	>20
	Vanceril Double Strength	84	2 to 6	6 to 10	>10
Triamcinolone	Azmacort	100	4 to 10	10 to 20	>20
Flunisolide	AeroBid	250	2 to 4	4 to 8	>8
Fluticasone	Flovent 44	44	2 to 6		
	Flovent 110	110	2	2 to 6	>6
	Flovent 220	220			>3

Drug	Trade name	Dose (μg/puff)	Dose range (total puffs/day)		
			Low	Intermediate	High
Mast cell stabilizers					
Cromolyn sodium MDI	Intal	800 mg/puff nebulizer, 20 mg/2-mL ampule	Adults: 6 puffs or 3 ampules in three divided doses Children: 3 puffs or 3 ampules in three divided doses	Adults: 9 to 12 puffs in three divided doses Children: 6 puffs in three divided doses	Adults: 16 puffs in three divided doses or 4 ampules in four divided doses Children: 8 puffs or 4 ampules in four divided doses
Nedocromil	Tilade	1.75 mg/puff	Adults: 4 to 6 puffs in two to three divided doses Children: 2 to 3 puffs in two to three divided doses	Adults: 9 to 12 puffs in two to three divided doses Children: 4 to 6 puffs in two to three divided doses	Adults: 16 puffs in four divided doses Children: 8 puffs in four divided doses

2. **Cromolyn sodium (Intal, Nasalcrom) and nedocromil sodium (Tilade)** are anti-inflammatory medications. They lack the systemic side effects associated with corticosteroids. Cromolyn, available in a metered-dose inhaler or as inhaler solution, requires dosing four times per day. Nedocromil is designed for twice-daily dosing. Maximal benefit may not be achieved for four to six weeks. Cromolyn and nedocromil are first-line agents in children.

3. **Leukotriene modifiers**
   a. **Zafirlukast (Accolate), montelukast (Singulair) and zileuton (Zyflo)** interfere with the actions of leukotriene inflammatory mediators, preventing bronchoconstriction. Zileuton is a 5-lipoxygenase inhibitor. Zafirlukast is a leukotriene receptor antagonist. Montelukast is similar to zafirlukast but is taken only once per day at night. Zafirlukast must be taken on an empty stomach.
   b. Zafirlukast and zileuton may interfere with the metabolism of warfarin (Coumadin).
   c. Zileuton has been associated with elevated levels of liver enzymes; thus, periodic monitoring of alanine transaminase is required. Zafirlukast (Accolate, 20 mg bid, on an empty stomach), montelukast (Singular, 10 mg PO qhs) and zileuton (Zyflo, 600 mg PO qid) are alternatives for patients with mild persistent asthma who are not candidates for inhaled anti-inflammatory medications.

4. **Long-acting beta$_2$ agonists.** If inhaled anti-inflammatory medications do not prevent asthma symptoms, an inhaled long-acting beta$_2$ agonist may be added. Long-acting beta$_2$ agonists relax bronchial smooth muscle. Salmeterol (Serevent, 2 puffs bid), a long-acting beta$_2$ agonist, has a slower onset of action (up to 30 minutes) but a longer duration (at least 12 hours) than short-acting beta$_2$ agonists. Salmeterol improves nighttime and exercise-associated symptoms. Patients should not use salmeterol for acute asthma attacks.

5. **Methylxanthines** use has declined with the arrival of safer and more

effective medications. However, they still have a role in asthma therapy when newer anti-inflammatory medications fail to provide relief. Theophylline produces smooth muscle relaxation resulting in bronchodilation but also improves diaphragmatic contractility and increases mucociliary clearance. It may also have some anti-inflammatory effects. Selected patients may benefit from a sustained-action theophylline preparation in the evening, with the drug titrated to a serum concentration ranging from 5 to 15 µg/mL. Theophylline sustained release (Theo-Dur, 100-400 mg PO bid).

Beta$_2$ Agonists and Dosing		
Drug	Trade name	Dosage
Long-Acting Agent		
Salmeterol	Serevent	2 puffs bid
Short-Acting Agents		
Albuterol	Ventolin Rotacaps Proventil Ventolin	One inhaled capsule every four to eight hours prn 2-4 puffs q4-8h prn
Albuterol HTA	Proventil HFA	2-4 puffs q4-8h prn
Bitolterol	Tornalate	2-4 puffs q4-8h prn
Pirbuterol	Maxair	2-4 puffs q4-8h prn

C. Quick-relief medications
   1. **Short-acting beta$_2$ agonists** are rescue medications which should only be used as monotherapy in patients with mild and intermittent asthma. These potent bronchodilators provide quick relief of acute symptoms.
   2. **Anticholinergics.** Ipratropium (Atrovent) reverses bronchospasm and may have an additive effect when used with inhaled short-acting beta$_2$ agonists.
   3. **Systemic corticosteroids.** In patients with moderate to severe exacerbations of asthma, use of systemic corticosteroids during an attack can prevent further progression of the episode. Seven to 10 days is usually sufficient. Prednisone, prednisolone or methylprednisolone, 40 to 60 mg qd. The oral steroid does not have to be tapered after a short-course of therapy if the patient is on an inhaled steroid.

III. Management of acute exacerbations
   A. High-dose, short-acting beta$_2$ agonists delivered by a metered-dose inhaler with a volume spacer or via a nebulizer remain the mainstays of urgent treatment. Nebulized ipratropium bromide may enhance the bronchodilation provided by a short-acting beta$_2$ agonist. Supplemental oxygen should be used to maintain the oxygen saturation at greater than 90 percent.
   B. Most patients require therapy with systemic corticosteroids to resolve symptoms and prevent relapse.
   C. Hospitalization should be considered if the PEFR remains less than 70% of predicted. Patients with a PEFR less than 50% of predicted who exhibit an increasing pCO_2 level and declining mental status are candidates for intubation.

References: See page 195.

Chronic Obstructive Pulmonary Disease

Chronic obstructive pulmonary disease is the fourth leading cause of death. Emphysema and chronic bronchitis are the main disease states that comprise chronic obstructive pulmonary disease, although there is usually significant overlap between the two conditions.

I. **Pathogenesis**
   A. **Emphysema** is characterized by permanent enlargement of the alveolar air spaces with destruction of the alveolar walls.
   B. **Chronic bronchitis** is defined as chronic sputum production and variable degrees of airway obstruction for more than 3 months in each of 3 successive years.
   C. **Smoking** is the single overwhelming risk factor for the development of COPD. Pipe and cigar smokers are at intermediate risk for COPD.

II. **Diagnosis of chronic obstructive pulmonary disease**
   A. **Symptoms** are often insidious and may be manifest early by exercise intolerance. Later symptoms include wheezing, dyspnea, chronic cough, sputum production, recurrent pneumonias, and bronchitis.
   B. **Signs.** Wheezing, decreased air movement in the chest, hyperinflation, prolonged expiratory time, barrel chest and supraclavicular retractions are characteristic.
   C. **Pulmonary function testing**
      1. Significant airway obstruction is present when the forced expiratory volume in 1 sec (FEV_1) is less than 80% of predicted, and the FEV_1/Forced Vital Capacity ratio is less than 70% of predicted.
      2. Hyperinflated lungs are indicated by an increased total lung capacity and residual volume and by loss of alveolar surface area and decreased diffusing capacity.

III. **Management of chronic obstructive pulmonary disease**
   A. **Smoking cessation** is effective in halting the progression of chronic obstructive pulmonary disease.
   B. **Ipratropium bromide (Atrovent)**
      1. These drugs are first-line agents for COPD. Ipratropium may produce bronchodilation and can reduce sputum volume without altering viscosity. It should be used regularly with a beta agonist for most patients with COPD.
      2. 4-6 puffs qid or 2.5 mL (500 mcg) nebulized qid.
   C. **Beta-agonists**
      1. **Beta2-adrenergic agonists** should be used for "as needed" treatment for symptom relief. Side effects include tremor, nervousness, tachycardia, and hypokalemia in high doses.
      2. **Dosages**
         a. **Albuterol (Ventolin)** MDI, 2-4 puffs qid prn, or powder 200 mcg/capsule inhaled qid prn.
         b. **Bitolterol (Tornalate)** MDI, 2-4 puffs qid prn.
         c. **Salmeterol (Serevent)** MDI, 2 puffs bid; long-acting agent; useful for nocturnal symptoms; not effective for acute exacerbations.
   D. **Theophylline**
      1. Theophylline has utility in patients with significant side effects from high dose beta agonists as well as in patients with nocturnal symptoms. It has been shown to improve airflow, decrease dyspnea, and improve ventilation, arterial blood gases, exercise tolerance, and respiratory muscle function.
      2. It should be used after adequate doses of ipratropium and beta2-agonists

have been tried. A dosage that yields a serum drug level ranging from 8 to 12 ug/mL is recommended. Evening dosing may control decreased nighttime airflows and improve morning respiratory symptoms. Adverse drug interactions occur with ciprofloxacin, erythromycin, cimetidine, and zileuton.

3. **Dosage of long-acting theophylline.** 200-300 mg bid. Theophylline preparations with 24 hour action may be administered once a day in the early evening. Theo-24, 100-400 mg qd [100, 200, 300, 400 mg].

E. Corticosteroids

1. Corticosteroids produce a favorable response during acute COPD exacerbations, improving symptoms and reducing the length of hospitalization. Short courses of corticosteroids should be considered in patients with acute exacerbations who are unresponsive to aggressive inhaled bronchodilator therapy.

2. Long-term use of corticosteroids should be considered only in patients who have continued symptoms or severe airflow limitation despite maximal therapy with other agents. Only 20% to 30% of patients show objective benefits from long-term corticosteroid administration.

3. Aerosolized corticosteroids provide the benefits of oral corticosteroids with fewer side effects.
   Triamcinolone (Azmacort) MDI 2-4 puffs bid.
   Flunisolide (Aerobid, Aerobid-M) MDI 2-4 puffs bid.
   Beclomethasone (Beclovent) MDI 2-5 puffs bid.
   Budesonide (Pulmicort) MDI 2 puffs bid.

4. Oral steroids are warranted in severe COPD. Prednisone 0.5-1.0 mg/kg or 40 mg qAM. The dose should be tapered over 1-2 weeks following clinical improvement.

5. **Side effects of corticosteroids.** Cataracts, osteoporosis, sodium and water retention, hypokalemia, muscle weakness, aseptic necrosis of femoral and humeral heads, peptic ulcer disease, pancreatitis, endocrine and skin abnormalities, muscle wasting.

IV. Surgical treatment. Lung volume reduction surgery (LVRS) consists of surgical removal of an emphysematous bulla. This procedure can ameliorate symptoms and improve pulmonary function. Lung transplantation is reserved for those patients deemed unsuitable or too ill for LVRS. It is effective for severe emphysema.

V. Treatment of complications of COPD

A. Infection

1. Infection frequently causes bronchitis exacerbations and is associated with increased or purulent sputum, increased cough, chest congestion and discomfort, and increased dyspnea and wheezing. Chills and fever suggest pneumonia. Acute bacterial episodes tend to be seasonal, appearing more frequently in the winter.

2. **Gram stain**
   a. Gram stain is a useful guide in the selection of an empiric antibiotic. The presence of more than 25 neutrophils and fewer than 10 epithelial cells per low-power field indicates that the specimen is sputum.
   b. The presence of bacteria on high-power examination of such a specimen is presumptive evidence of infection. Although patients with COPD may be colonized by Hemophilus influenzae and Streptococcus pneumoniae, these organisms should not be present in sufficient numbers to be seen on a Gram stain.

3. **Sputum culture and sensitivity** testing are generally not necessary but may be required if the patient is very ill or if the infection is hospital-acquired.

4. **A chest film** is helpful in ruling out pneumonia or other disorders.

5. **Pathogens for COPD exacerbations** include H. influenzae, parainfluenzae, S. pneumoniae, and Moraxella catarrhalis. Mycoplasma

pneumoniae or Chlamydia may be present. Other less common pathogens are staphylococci, Neisseria, Klebsiella, and Pseudomonas.

6. **Treatment of exacerbations of COPD**
   a. Treat for 10-14 days.
   b. Trimethoprim/Sulfamethoxazole (Septra DS) 160/800 mg PO bid.
   c. Amoxicillin/clavulanate (Augmentin) 500 mg tid or 875 mg PO bid [250, 500, 875 mg]; stable against beta lactamases; gastrointestinal side effects (diarrhea) are common.
   d. Cefuroxime axetil (Ceftin), 250-500 mg PO bid; good activity against primary pathogens; stable against beta lactamase.
   e. Cefixime (Suprax), 200 mg PO bid or 400 mg PO qd; stable against beta lactamase, lacks Staphylococcus aureus coverage.
   f. Azithromycin (Zithromax), 500 mg on day 1, then 250 mg PO qd; reserved for treatment of infections due to Mycoplasma, Chlamydia, Legionella species.
   g. Clarithromycin (Biaxin), 250-500 mg bid; moderate activity against H influenzae.
   h. Levofloxacin (Levaquin) 500 mg PO qd. Broad spectrum coverage.

7. **Preventive Care**
   a. **Immunization.** Pneumococcal vaccination every six years, and yearly influenza vaccinations should be provided.
   b. Influenza therapy should be considered when unimmunized patients are at high risk for contracting influenza or there is inadequate time for immunization. Amantadine (Symmetrel) 100 mg PO bid (qd if >65 years old). Rimantadine (Flumadine) 100 mg PO bid (qd if >65 years old).

B. **Hypoxemia**. Hypoxemia adversely affects function and increases risk of death, and oxygen therapy is the only treatment documented to improve survival in patients with COPD. Oxygen is usually delivered by nasal cannula at a flow rate sufficient to maintain an optimal oxygen saturation level.

References: See page 195.

Infectious Diseases

Community-acquired Pneumonia

Community-acquired pneumonia affects about 4 million patients each year. About 20% of these cases require hospitalization, the condition. Mortality rates range from 1% to 5% in outpatients and from 15% to 30% in inpatients, making it the sixth leading cause of death.

I. **Pathophysiology**
   A. Pathogens in community-acquired pneumonia include Streptococcus pneumoniae (33%), Haemophilus influenzae (10%), Legionella species (7%), and Chlamydia pneumoniae (5%) Other organisms include Mycoplasma pneumoniae, other gram-positive organisms, gram-negative organisms, anaerobes, mycobacteria, fungi, and viruses. S pneumoniae is the leading cause of community-acquired pneumonia in both inpatients and outpatients.
   B. **Factors that increase susceptibility to pneumonia** include age over 65 years, the presence of chronic underlying illness, and certain local epidemiologic. More than half of cases occur in patients over age 65
   C. **Factors that increase risk of death**
      1. Age over 65 also increases the risk of death from community-acquired pneumonia. Additional risk factors for death from this condition include the following:
         a. Multilobar, necrotizing, aspiration, or postobstructive infection
         b. Abnormal vital signs, particularly a respiratory rate of 30 breaths/minute or more, pulse of 125 beats/minute or more, systolic blood pressure less than 90 mm Hg, and decreased (<95°F [<35°C]) or elevated (>104°F [>40°C]) temperature
         c. Abnormal laboratory findings, particularly a low (<4,000/mm^3) or high (>30,000/mm^3) white blood cell count, hypoxemia or hypercapnia, anemia, elevated blood urea nitrogen level, or elevated creatinine level
         d. Altered mental status
         e. Presence of neoplastic disease
         f. Presence of comorbid disease involving the immune, lung, endocrine, renal, cardiac, liver, or reticuloendothelial system
         g. History of alcohol abuse and malnutrition
         h. Evidence of extrapulmonary sites of involvement
         i. Multiorgan infection

II. **Clinical evaluation**
   A. Outpatient treatment of community-acquired pneumonia is largely empirical. All patients should have a chest film taken, since a diagnosis of pneumonia cannot be established in the absence of infiltrates. Patients who have physical findings consistent with pneumonia but negative findings on chest films should be treated as though they have pneumonia.
   B. Vital signs should be evaluated and a complete blood cell count should be taken, since certain abnormal values are independent predictors of increased mortality. Sputum and blood culture and sputum Gram's stain should usually be reserved for patients who are sick enough to need hospitalization.

Oral Antibiotic Regimens for Community-acquired Pneumonia	
Drug	**Recommended regimen**
Erythromycin	500 mg q6h
Clarithromycin (Biaxin)	500 mg q12h
Azithromycin (Zithromax)	Day 1,500 mg; then 250 mg qd
Levofloxacin (Levaquin)	500 mg qd
Sparfloxacin (Zagam)	Day 1,400 mg; then 200 mg qd
Trovafloxacin (Trovan)	200 mg qd
Grepafloxacin (Raxar)	600 mg qd
Doxycycline	100 mg bid

III. Outpatient therapy for community-acquired pneumonia
    A. Antibiotics should be chosen that provide adequate coverage against the presumed organisms known to cause community-acquired pneumonia. A macrolide is recommended, including erythromycin, clarithromycin (Biaxin), or azithromycin (Zithromax); the fluoroquinolones levofloxacin (Levaquin), trovafloxacin mesylate (Trovan), grepafloxacin (Raxar), sparfloxacin (Zagam), and any other fluoroquinolone with enhanced activity against S pneumoniae; and (in patients between the ages of 17 and 40) doxycycline.

    B. Duration of therapy should be 7 to 10 days.

References: See page 195.

Sinusitis

Sinusitis affects 12% of adults and complicates 0.5% of viral upper respiratory infections. Symptoms that have been present for less than 1 month are indicative of acute sinusitis, while symptoms of longer duration reflect chronic sinusitis.

I. Pathophysiology
    A. Factors that predispose to sinus infection include anatomic abnormalities, viral URIs, allergies, overuse of topical decongestants, asthma, and immune deficiencies.

    B. Acute sinusitis is associated with the same bacteria as otitis media. Streptococcus pneumoniae, Hemophilus influenzae, and Moraxella catarrhalis are the most commonly encountered pathogens. Thirty five percent of H influenzae and 75% of M catarrhalis strains produce beta-lactamases, making them resistant to penicillin antibiotics.

    C. Chronic sinusitis is associated with Staphylococcus aureus and anaerobes.

II. Clinical evaluation
    A. If symptoms have lasted for less than 7 to 10 days and the patient is recovering, a self-limited viral URI is the most likely cause. However, worsening symptoms or symptoms that persist for more than 7 days are

more likely to be caused by sinusitis.

B. Symptoms of acute sinusitis include facial pain or tenderness, nasal congestion, purulent nasal and postnasal discharge, headache, maxillary tooth pain, malodorous breath, fever, and eye swelling. Pain or pressure in the cheeks and deep nasal recesses is common.

C. High fever and signs of acute toxicity are unusual except in the most severe cases. Purulent drainage in the patient's nose or throat may sometimes be seen.

D. The nasal mucosa is often erythematous and swollen. The presence of mucopus in the external nares or posterior pharynx is highly suggestive of sinusitis. Facial tenderness, elicited by percussion, is an unreliable sign of sinusitis.

III. Laboratory evaluation

A. **Imaging.** Plain films are usually unnecessary for evaluating acute sinusitis because of the high cost and relative insensitivity.

B. **CT scanning** is useful if the diagnosis remains uncertain or if orbital or intracranial complications are suspected. CT scanning is nonspecific and may demonstrate sinus abnormalities in 87% of patients with colds.

C. **MRI** is useful when fungal infections or tumors are seriously considered.

D. **Sinus aspiration** is an invasive procedure, and is only indicated for complicated sinusitis, immunocompromise, failure to respond to multiple courses of empiric antibiotic therapy, or severe symptoms.

E. Cultures of nasal secretions correlate poorly with results of sinus aspiration.

IV. Management of sinusitis

A. **Antibiotic therapy for sinusitis**

1. **First-line agents**

   a. Amoxicillin (Amoxil): Adults, 500 mg tid PO for 14 days. Children, 40 mg/kg/d in 3 divided doses.

   b. Trimethoprim/sulfamethoxazole (Bactrim, Septra): Adults, 1 DS tab (160/800 mg) bid. Children, 8/40 mg/kg/d bid.

   c. Erythromycin/sulfisoxazole (Pediazole): Children, 50/150 mg/kg/d qid.

2. A 2-3 week course of therapy is recommended; however, if the patient is improved but still symptomatic at the end of the course, the medication should be continued for an additional 5 to 7 days after symptoms subside.

3. **Broader-spectrum agents**

   a. If the initial response to antibiotics is unsatisfactory, beta-lactamase-producing bacteria are likely to be present, and broad-spectrum therapy is required.

   b. Amoxicillin/clavulanate (Augmentin): adults, 250 mg tid or 875 mg bid; children, 40 mg/kg/d in 3 divided doses.

   c. Cefuroxime axetil (Ceftin): adults, 250 mg bid; children, 125 mg bid.

   d. Cefixime (Suprax): adults, 200 mg bid; children, 8 mg/kg/d bid.

   e. Cefpodoxime (Vantin) 200 mg bid

   f. Loracarbef (Lorabid): 400 mg bid.

   g. Azithromycin (Zithromax): 500 mg as a single dose on day 1, then 250 mg qd.

   h. Clarithromycin (Biaxin): 500 mg bid.

4. **Penicillin-resistant S. Pneumoniae** result from bacterial alterations in penicillin-binding proteins. Highly resistant strains are resistant to penicillin, trimethoprim/sulfamethoxazole (TMP/SMX), and third-generation cephalosporins. The prevalence of multiple-drug resistant S. pneumoniae is 20-35%. High dose amoxicillin (80 mg/kg/d), or amoxicillin plus amoxicillin/clavulanate, or clindamycin are options.

B. **Chronic sinusitis** is commonly caused by anaerobic organisms. 3-4 weeks of therapy or longer is required.

C. **Ancillary treatments**

1. **Steam and saline** improves drainage of mucus. Spray saline (NaSal)

or a bulb syringe with a saline solution (1 tsp of salt in 1 qt of warm water) may be used.

    2. **Decongestants**
        a. Topical or systemic decongestants may be used in acute or chronic sinusitis, including phenylephrine (Neo-Synephrine) or oxymetazoline (Afrin) nasal drops or sprays.
        b. Oral decongestants, such as phenylephrine or pseudoephedrine, are active in areas not reached by topical agents.

References: See page 195.

Tonsillopharyngitis

In about a quarter of patients with a sore throat, the disorder is caused by group A beta-hemolytic streptococcus. Treatment of streptococcal tonsillopharyngitis reduces the occurrence of subsequent rheumatic fever, an inflammatory disease that affects the joints and heart and sometimes the skin, central nervous system, and subcutaneous tissues.

I. **Prevalence of pharyngitis**
    A. Group A beta-hemolytic streptococcus (GABHS) typically occurs in patients 5-11 years of age, and it is uncommon in children under 3 years old. Most cases of GABHS occur in late winter and early spring.
    B. **Etiologic causes of sore throat**
        1. **Viral.** Rhinoviruses, influenza, Epstein-Barr virus.
        2. **Bacterial.** GABHS (Streptococcus pyogenes), Streptococcus pneumoniae, Haemophilus influenzae, Moraxella catarrhalis, Staphylococcus aureus, anaerobes, Mycoplasma pneumoniae, Candida albicans.
    C. In patients who present with pharyngitis, the major goal is to detect GABHS infection because rheumatic fever may result. Severe GABHS infections may also cause a toxic-shock-like illness (toxic strep syndrome), bacteremia, streptococcal deep tissue infections (necrotizing fasciitis), and streptococcal cellulitis.

II. **Clinical Evaluation of Sore Throat**
    A. GABHS infection is characterized by sudden onset of sore throat, fever and tender swollen anterior cervical lymph nodes, typically in a child 5-11 years of age. Headache, nausea and vomiting may occur.
    B. Cough, rhinorrhea and hoarseness are generally absent.

III. **Physical examination**
    A. Streptococcal infection is suggested by erythema and swelling of the pharynx, enlarged and erythematous tonsils, tonsillar exudate, or palatal petechiae.
    B. Unilateral inflammation and swelling of the pharynx suggests peritonsillar abscess. Distortion of the posterior pharyngeal wall suggests a retropharyngeal abscess. Corynebacterium diphtheriae is indicated by a dull membrane which bleeds on manipulation. Viral infections may cause oral vesicular eruptions.
    C. The tympanic membranes should be examined for erythema or a middle ear effusion. Purulent nasal discharge, especially from the middle meatus, implies sinusitis. Tender lymph node enlargement usually occurs in an acute infection, whereas nontender enlargement is indicative of chronic infection or tumors.
    D. The lungs should be auscultated because viral infection occasionally causes pneumonia.
    E. The clinical diagnosis of GABHS infection is correct in only 50-75% of cases when based on clinical criteria alone.

IV. **Diagnostic testing**
    A. **Rapid streptococcal testing** has a specificity of 90% and a sensitivity of

80%. A dry swab should be used to sample both the posterior wall and the tonsillar fossae, especially erythematous or exudative areas.

B. Throat culture is the most accurate test available for the diagnosis of GABHS pharyngitis.

C. Diagnostic approach
1. Patients presenting with an acute episode of pharyngitis should receive a rapid streptococcal antigen test. If the rapid test is negative, a culture should be done.
2. If the rapid test is positive, treatment with an antibiotic should be initiated for 10 days. The presence of physical and historical findings suggesting GABHS infection may also prompt the initiation of antibiotic therapy despite a negative rapid strep test.
3. After throat culture, presumptive therapy should be initiated. If the culture is positive for GABHS, a 10-day course of therapy should be completed. If the culture is negative, antibiotics may be discontinued.

V. Antibiotic therapy
A. Starting antibiotic therapy within the first 24-48 hours of illness decreases the duration of sore throat, fever and adenopathy by 12-24 hours. Treatment also minimizes risk of transmission and of rheumatic fever.

B. Penicillin VK is the antibiotic of choice for GABS; 250 mg PO qid or 500 mg PO bid x 10 days [250, 500 mg]. A 10-day regimen is recommended. Penicillin G benzathine (Bicillin LA) may be used as one-time therapy when compliance is a concern; 1.2 million units IM x 1 dose.

C. Azithromycin (Zithromax) offers the advantage of once-a-day dosing for just 5 days; 500 mg x 1, then 250 mg qd x 4 days.

D. Clarithromycin (Biaxin), 500 mg PO bid; bacteriologic efficacy is similar to that of penicillin VK, and it may be taken twice a day.

E. Erythromycin is also effective; 250 mg PO qid; or enteric coated delayed release tablet (PCE) 333 mg PO tid or 500 mg PO bid [250, 333, 500 mg]. **Erythromycin ethyl succinate (EES)** 400 PO qid or 800 mg PO bid [400 mg]. Gastrointestinal upset is common.

VI. Treatment of recurrent GABHS pharyngitis
A. When patient compliance is an issue, an injection of penicillin G benzathine may be appropriate. When patient compliance is not an issue, therapy should be changed to a broader spectrum agent.
1. **Cephalexin (Keflex)** 250-500 mg tid x 5 days [250, 500 mg]
2. **Cefadroxil (Duricef)** 500 mg bid x 5 days [500 mg]
3. **Loracarbef (Lorabid)** 200-400 mg bid x 5 days [200, 400 mg]
4. **Cefixime (Suprax)** 400 mg qd x 5 days [200, 400 mg]
5. **Ceftibuten (Cedax)** 400 mg qd x 5 days [400 mg]
6. **Cefuroxime axetil (Ceftin)** 250-500 mg bid x 5 days [125, 250, 500 mg]

B. Amoxicillin/clavulanate (Augmentin) has demonstrated superior results in comparison with penicillin; 250-500 mg tid or 875 mg bid [250, 500, 875 mg].

C. Sulfonamides, trimethoprim, and the tetracyclines are not effective for the treatment of GABHS pharyngitis.

References: See page 195.

Primary Care of HIV-Infected Adults

I. Initial evaluation
A. The initial evaluation of the HIV-infected adult should include an assessment of the patient's past medical history, current symptoms and treatments, a complete physical examination, and laboratory testing.

B. Previous conditions
1. Prior medical conditions related to HIV infection should be assessed.

Mucocutaneous candidiasis, oral hairy leukoplakia, hepatitis, pneumonia, sexually transmitted diseases, and tuberculosis should be sought. Past episodes of varicella-zoster, herpes simplex virus lesions, and opportunistic infections should be assessed.

2. Dates and results of earlier tuberculin skin tests should be obtained. Women should be are asked about dates and results of Pap smears. Previous immunizations and antiretroviral therapy should be documented.

C. **Current conditions and symptoms.** Fever, night sweats, unexplained weight loss, lymphadenopathy, oral discomfort, visual changes, unusual headaches, swallowing difficulties, diarrhea, dermatologic conditions, and respiratory and neurologic symptoms are suggestive of opportunistic infections or a malignant process.

D. **Social history** includes information on past and present drug use, sexual behavior, dietary habits, household pets, employment, and current living situation. Residence and travel history should be assessed because coccidioidomycosis and histoplasmosis are more common in certain geographic regions.

II. **Physical examination**

A. Weight, temperature, skin, oropharynx, fundi, lymph nodes, lungs, abdominal organs, genitalia, rectum, and the nervous system should be assessed. A cervical Pap smear should be obtained from women who have not had a normal result in the past year.

B. Screening for Neisseria gonorrhoeae and chlamydial infection should be considered for sexually active men and women.

III. **Laboratory tests**

A. **Complete blood count, chemistry profile, and serologic studies** for syphilis (rapid plasma reagin or VDRL), Toxoplasma gondii (IgG antibody), and hepatitis B (surface antigen, core antibody) should be obtained.

B. Patients should have a tuberculin skin test unless they have been reactive in the past or have been treated for the disease. In HIV-infected persons, a positive test is 5 mm or more of induration.

C. **A baseline chest film** is useful because many opportunistic pulmonary infections present with very subtle radiographic findings. A chest radiograph may suggest unrecognized tuberculosis.

D. **CD4+ counts** assist in determination of the degree of immunologic damage, assess risk of opportunistic complications, and guide the use of prophylaxis against infections.

E. **HIV RNA levels**

1. Quantitation of plasma HIV RNA (viral load), a marker of the rate of viral replication, is useful in determining prognosis. It is used to estimate the risk of disease progression and to aid in making antiretroviral therapy decisions.

2. HIV RNA levels generally vary no more than 0.3 log in clinically stable patients. Sustained changes greater than threefold (0.5 log) are significant. A decrease occurs with successful antiretroviral therapy. An upward trend in a patient not receiving antiretroviral therapy indicates an increase in viral replication. Increases noted during treatment suggest antiretroviral drug failure or poor adherence.

Treatment Goals for HIV RNA Levels	
Parameter	**Recommendation**
Target level of HIV RNA after initiation of treatment	Undetectable; <5,000 copies/mL

Parameter	Recommendation
Minimal decrease in HIV RNA indicative of antiretroviral activity	>0.5 log decrease
Change in HIV RNA that suggests drug treatment failure	Rise in HIV RNA level Failure to achieve desired reduction in HIV RNA level
Suggested frequency of HIV RNA measurement	At baseline: 2 measurements, 2-4 wk apart. 3-4 wk after initiating or changing therapy Every 3-4 mo in conjunction with CD4+ counts

3. HIV RNA levels should be obtained before the initiation or change of antiretroviral therapy. The next determination should be done a month after therapeutic intervention to assess its effect and then every 3 or 4 months.
4. Quantitative HIV RNA assays include branched DNA (bDNA) (Multiplex) and reverse transcriptase-initiated polymerase chain reaction (RT-PCR) (Amplicor HIV-1 Monitor). While both tests provide similar information, concentrations of HIV RNA obtained with the RT-PCR test are about twofold higher than those obtained by the bDNA method. For this reason, all HIV RNA determinations in a single patient should be obtained using the same assay.

IV. Prevention of infections
A. Vaccinations
1. Vaccination with pneumococcal vaccine, polyvalent (Pneumovax 23, Pnu-Immune 23) is recommended when HIV infection is diagnosed. Yearly influenza vaccination is suggested. Those who are seronegative for hepatitis B and at risk for infection should be offered hepatitis B vaccine (Recombivax HB, Engerix-B).
2. Tetanus vaccine should be administered every 10 years, and hepatitis A vaccine (Havrix, Vaqta) should be considered for nonimmune sexually active patients.

B. Opportunistic infections
1. **Pneumocystis carinii pneumonia** is rarely encountered in patients receiving prophylactic therapy. Indications for prophylaxis are a CD4+ count below 200 cells/μL, HIV-related thrush, or unexplained fever for 2 or more weeks regardless of CD4+ count. Anyone with a past history of PCP should continue suppressive therapy indefinitely because of the high risk of relapse.
2. **Toxoplasmosis** risk increases as the CD4+ count approaches 100 cells/μL, and patients who are seropositive for IgG antibody to toxoplasma should begin preventive therapy when the count nears this level. Patients who have been treated for toxoplasmosis require lifelong suppressive therapy.

USPHS/IDSA Guidelines for Prevention of Opportunistic Infections in HIV-Infected Patients

Pathogen	Indication for prophylaxis	First-choice drug	Selected alternative drugs
Prophylaxis Strongly Recommended			
Pneumocystis carinii	CD4+ count <200 cells/μL or unexplained fever for >2 wk or oropharyngeal candidiasis	TMP-SMX (Bactrim, Septra), 1 DS tablet PO daily	Dapsone, 100 mg PO daily, or aerosolized pentamidine (NebuPent), 300 mg monthly
Mycobacterium tuberculosis	Tuberculin skin test reaction of >5 mm or prior positive test without treatment or exposure to active tuberculosis	Isoniazid, 300 mg PO, plus pyridoxine, 50 mg PO daily for 12 mo	Rifampin, 600 mg PO daily for 12 mo
Toxoplasma gondii	IgG antibody to T gondii and CD4+ count <100 cells/μL	TMP-SMX, 1 DS tablet PO daily	Dapsone, 50 mg PO daily, plus pyrimethamine (Daraprim), 50 mg PO weekly, plus leucovorin (Wellcovorin), 25 mg PO weekly
Mycobacterium avium complex	CD4+ <50 cells/μL	Clarithromycin (Biaxin), 500 mg PO bid, or azithromycin (Zithromax), 1,200 mg PO weekly	Rifabutin (Mycobutin), 300 mg PO daily
Streptococcus pneumoniae	All patients	Pneumococcal vaccine (Pneumovax 23, Pnu-Immune 23), 0.5 mL IM once	None
Consideration of Prophylaxis Recommended			
Hepatitis B virus	All seronegative patients	Hepatitis B vaccine (Engerix-B, 20 pg IM x 3, or Recombivax HB, 10 μg IM x 3)	None
Influenza virus	All patients, annually before influenza season	0.5 mL IM	Rimantadine (Flumadine), 100 mg PO bid, or amantadine (Symadine, Symmetrel), 100 mg PO bid

C. **Tuberculosis**. Patients who have HIV infection and positive results on tuberculin skin tests have a 2-10% per year risk of reactivation. If active tuberculosis has been excluded, prophylaxis should be prescribed to

HIV-infected patients who have a tuberculin skin test reaction of 5 mm or more, who have a history of a positive tuberculin skin test reaction but were never treated, or who have had close contact with someone with active tuberculosis.

D. **Mycobacterium avium complex infection.** Prophylactic therapy is recommended for patients whose CD4+ counts are less than 50 cells/μL. Azithromycin (Zithromax), 1,200 mg (2 tabs) weekly by mouth is recommended.

E. **Antiretroviral therapy**
   1. Antiretroviral drug regimens may suppress HIV replication almost completely in some patients. These changes are associated with improved survival and a lengthening in the time to development of AIDS-defining conditions.
   2. HIV RNA levels are used to identify those patients who are at greatest risk for progression of disease and likely to benefit from antiretroviral therapy. HIV RNA quantitation also documents treatment efficacy and failure.

Antiretroviral Therapy

Initiate therapy for patients with:
   Symptomatic HIV disease
   Asymptomatic HIV disease but CD4+ count <500 cells/μL
   HIV RNA levels >5,000 to 10,000 copies/mL

Consider therapy for patients with:
   Detectable HIV RNA levels who request it and are committed to lifelong adherence

Recommended initial regimens:
   2 NRTIs and 1 protease inhibitor
      Zidovudine (AZT, Retrovir) + lamivudine (3TC, Epivir), didanosine (ddI, Videx), or zalcitabine (ddC, Hivid) + potent protease inhibitor or
      Stavudine (d4T, Zerit) + lamivudine or didanosine + potent protease inhibitor
   2 NRTIs and 1 NNRTI
      Zidovudine (AZT, Retrovir) + lamivudine, didanosine, or zalcitabine + nevirapine (Viramune) or delavirdine mesylate (Rescriptor) or
      Stavudine + lamivudine or didanosine + nevirapine or delavirdine

Change therapy for:
   Treatment failure, as indicated by
      Rising HIV RNA level
      Failure to achieve target decrease in HIV RNA
      Declining CD4+ count
      Clinical progression
   Toxicity, intolerance, or nonadherance

References: See page 195.

Diverticulitis

By age 50, one third of adults have diverticulosis coli; two thirds have diverticulosis by age 80. Ten to 20% of patients with diverticulosis will have diverticulitis or diverticular hemorrhage. Causes of diverticulosis include aging, elevation of colonic intraluminal pressure, and decreased dietary fiber. Eighty-five percent are found in the sigmoid colon.

I. **Clinical presentation of diverticulitis**
   A. Diverticulitis is characterized by the abrupt onset of unremitting left-lower quadrant abdominal pain, fever, and an alteration in bowel pattern. Diverticulitis of the transverse colon may simulate ulcer pain; diverticulitis of the cecum and redundant sigmoid may resemble appendicitis. Frank rectal bleeding is usually not seen with diverticulitis.
   B. **Physical exam.** Left-lower quadrant tenderness is characteristic. Abdominal examination is often deceptively unremarkable in the elderly and in persons taking corticosteroids.

Differential Diagnosis of Diverticulitis	
Elderly	**Middle Aged and Young**
Ischemic colitis	Appendicitis
Carcinoma	Salpingitis
Volvulus	Inflammatory bowel disease
Colonic Obstruction	Penetrating ulcer
Penetrating ulcer	Urosepsis
Nephrolithiasis/urosepsis	

II. **Diagnostic evaluation**
   A. **Plain X-rays** may show ileus, obstruction, mass effect, ischemia, or perforation.
   B. **CT scan** is the test of choice to evaluate acute diverticulitis. The CT scan can be used for detecting complications and ruling out other diseases.
   C. **Contrast enema.** Water soluble contrast is safe and useful in mild-to-moderate cases of diverticulitis when the diagnosis is in doubt.
   D. **Endoscopy.** Acute diverticulitis is a relative contraindication to endoscopy; perforation should be excluded first. Endoscopy is indicated when the diagnosis is in doubt to exclude the possibility of ischemic bowel, Crohn's disease, or carcinoma.
   E. **Complete blood count** may show leukocytosis.

III. **Treatment**
   A. **Outpatient treatment**
      1. **Clear liquid diet**
      2. **Oral antibiotics**
         a. Ciprofloxacin (Cipro) 500 mg PO bid AND
         b. Metronidazole (Flagyl) 500 mg PO qid.
   B. **Inpatient treatment**
      1. Severe cases require hospitalization for gastrointestinal tract rest (NPO), intravenous fluid hydration, correction of electrolyte abnormalities, and antibiotics. Nasogastric suction is initiated if the patient is vomiting or if there is abdominal distention.
      2. Antibiotic coverage should include enteric gram-negative and anaerobic organisms
         a. Ampicillin 1-2 gm IV q4-6h **AND**
         b. Gentamicin or tobramycin 100-120 mg IV (1.5-2 mg/kg), then 80 mg IV q8h (5 mg/kg/d) **AND**

    c. Metronidazole (Flagyl) 500 mg IV q6-8h (15-30 mg/kg/d).
    d. Monotherapy with a second-generation cephalosporin (eg, cefoxitin, cefotetan) or an extended-spectrum penicillins (eg, piperacillin-tazobactam, ampicillin-sulbactam) also may be used.

C. The abdomen should be frequently reassessed for the first 48-72 hours. Improvement should occur over 48-72 hours, with decreased fever, leukocytosis, and abdominal pain. Failure to improve or deterioration are indications for reevaluation and consideration of surgery. Analgesics should be avoided because they may mask acute deterioration, and they may obscure the need for urgent operation.

D. Oral antibiotics should be continued for 1-2 weeks after resolution of the acute attack. Ciprofloxacin, 500 mg PO bid.

E. After the acute attack has resolved, clear liquids should be initiated, followed by a low residue diet for 1-2 weeks, followed by a high-fiber diet with psyllium.

IV. Surgical therapy
  A. An emergency sigmoid colectomy with proximal colostomy is indicated for attacks of diverticulitis associated with sepsis, peritonitis, obstruction, or perforation.
  B. Elective sigmoid resection is indicated for second or subsequent attacks of diverticulitis, or for attacks with complications managed nonoperatively (eg, percutaneous CT-guided drainage of an abscess), or carcinoma.
  C. Operative procedures
    1. Single stage procedure. This procedure is usually performed as an elective procedure after resolution of the acute attack of diverticulitis. The segment containing inflamed diverticulum (usually sigmoid colon) is resected with primary anastomosis. A bowel prep is required.
    2. Two stage procedure. This procedure is indicated for acute diverticulitis with obstruction or perforation with an unprepared bowel. The first stage consists of resection of the involved segment of colon, with end colostomy and either a mucous fistula or a Hartmann rectal pouch. The second stage consists of a colostomy take-down and reanastomosis after 2-3 months.

References: See page 195.

Urinary Tract Infection

An estimated 40 percent of women report having had a UTI at some point in their lives, and UTIs are the leading cause of gram-negative bacteremia.

I. Acute uncomplicated cystitis in young women
  A. Sexually active young women have the highest risk for UTIs. Their propensity to develop UTIs is caused by a short urethra, delays in micturition, sexual activity, and the use of diaphragms and spermicides.
  B. Symptoms of cystitis include dysuria, urgency, and frequency without fever or back pain. Lower tract infections are most common in women in their childbearing years. Fever is absent.
  C. A microscopic bacterial count of 100 CFU/mL of urine has a high positive predictive value for cystitis in symptomatic women. Ninety percent of uncomplicated cystitis episodes are caused by *Escherichia coli*, 10 to 20 percent are caused by coagulase-negative *Staphylococcus saprophyticus* and 5 percent are caused by other Enterobacteriaceae organisms or enterococci. Up to one-third of uropathogens are resistant to ampicillin, but the majority are susceptible to trimethoprim-sulfamethoxazole (85 to 95 percent) and fluoroquinolones (95 percent).
  D. Young women with acute uncomplicated cystitis should receive urinalysis (examination of spun urine), and a dipstick test for leukocyte esterase.

E. A positive leukocyte esterase test has a reported of 75 to 90 percent in detecting pyuria associated with a UTI. The dipstick test for nitrite indicates bacteriuria. Enterococci, *S. saprophyticus* and Acinetobacter species produce false-negative results on nitrite testing.

F. Three-day antibiotic regimens appear to offer the optimal combination of convenience, low cost and efficacy comparable to seven-day or longer regimens.

G. **Trimethoprim-sulfamethoxazole (Bactrim, Septra)**, 1 DS tab bid, remains the antibiotic of choice in the treatment of uncomplicated UTIs in young women.

H. The use of fluoroquinolones as first-line therapy for uncomplicated UTIs is recommended for patients who cannot tolerate sulfonamides or trimethoprim, who have a high frequency of antibiotic resistance because of recent antibiotic treatment, or who reside in an area with significant resistance to trimethoprim-sulfamethoxazole. Treatment should consist of a three-day regimens of one of the following:
   1. **Ciprofloxacin (Cipro)**, 250 mg bid.
   2. **Ofloxacin (Floxin)**, 200 mg bid.
   3. **Norfloxacin (Noroxin)** 400 mg bid.

I. A seven-day course should be considered in pregnant women, diabetic women and women who have had symptoms for more than one week and thus are at higher risk for pyelonephritis.

II. Recurrent cystitis in young women

A. Up to 20 percent of young women with acute cystitis develop recurrent UTIs. During these recurrent episodes, the causative organism should be identified by urine culture. Multiple infections caused by the same organism require longer courses of antibiotics and possibly further diagnostic tests. Most recurrent UTIs in young women are uncomplicated infections caused by different organisms. Women who have more than three UTI recurrences within one year can be managed using one of three preventive strategies:
   1. **Acute self-treatment** with a three-day course of standard therapy.
   2. **Postcoital prophylaxis** with one-half of a trimethoprim-sulfamethoxazole double-strength tablet (40/200 mg) if the UTIs have been clearly related to intercourse.
   3. **Continuous daily prophylaxis for six months:** Trimethoprim-sulfamethoxazole, one-half tablet/day (40/200 mg); norfloxacin (Noroxin), 200 mg/day; cephalexin (Keflex), 250 mg/day.

III. Pyelonephritis

A. Acute uncomplicated pyelonephritis presents with a mild cystitis-like illness and accompanying flank pain; fever, chills, nausea, vomiting, leukocytosis and abdominal pain; or a serious gram-negative bacteremia. The microbiologic features of acute uncomplicated pyelonephritis are the same as cystitis, except that *S. saprophyticus* is a rare cause.

B. The diagnosis should be confirmed by urinalysis with examination for pyuria and/or white blood cell casts and by urine culture. Urine cultures demonstrate more than 100,000 CFU/mL of urine. Blood cultures are positive in 20%. White cell casts are present on urinalysis.

C. Oral therapy should be considered in women with mild to moderate symptoms. Since *E. coli* resistance to ampicillin, amoxicillin and first-generation cephalosporins exceeds 30 percent in most locales, these agents should not be used for the treatment of pyelonephritis. Resistance to trimethoprim-sulfamethoxazole exceeds 15 percent; empiric therapy with ciprofloxacin (Cipro), 250 mg twice daily, or ofloxacin (Floxin), 200 mg twice daily, should be considered.

D. Patients who are too ill to take oral antibiotics should initially be treated parenterally with a third-generation cephalosporin, aztreonam, a broad-spectrum penicillin, a quinolone or an aminoglycoside. Once these patients have improved clinically (usually by day 3), they can be switched

to oral therapy
E. The total duration of therapy need is usually 14 days. Patients with persistent symptoms after three days of appropriate antimicrobial therapy should be evaluated by renal ultrasonography or computed tomography for evidence of urinary obstruction. In the small percentage of patients who relapse after a two-week course, a repeated six-week course is usually curative.

IV. Urinary tract infection in men
A. Urinary tract infections most commonly occur in older men with prostatic disease, outlet obstruction or urinary tract instrumentation. In men, a urine culture growing more than 1,000 CFU of a pathogen/mL of urine is the best sign of a urinary tract infection, with a sensitivity and specificity of 97 percent. Men with urinary tract infections should receive seven days of antibiotic therapy (trimethoprim-sulfamethoxazole or a fluoroquinolone).
B. Urologic evaluation should be performed routinely in adolescents and men with pyelonephritis or recurrent infections. When bacterial prostatitis is the source of a urinary tract infection, eradication usually requires antibiotic therapy for six to 12 weeks.

References: See page 195.

Herpes Simplex Virus Infections

Any mucocutaneous surface or visceral site may be infected by HSV. Two strains of the virus, herpes simplex virus type 1 (HSV-1) and herpes simplex virus type 2 (HSV-2), cause clinically indistinguishable lesions.

I. Pathogenesis of Herpes simplex
A. Both HSV-1 and HSV-2 may cause genital and orofacial lesions. In genital infections, recurrences are more commonly caused by HSV-2 than HSV-1.
B. Primary HSV infection occurs after first exposure, followed by a latency period while the virus remains dormant within the nerve ganglion. Antibody studies have shown that 60% of all US adults are positive for HSV antibody. The incubation period for primary HSV infections is 1-26 days.

II. Clinical features
A. Diagnostic features of HSV infection
1. The lesions consists of grouped vesicles or a solitary vesicle with erythematous bases, progressing to ulceration. Primary infections may be accompanied by flu-like symptoms.
2. Prodromal burning or itching is present in recurrent disease.
3. Lesions are painful and persist for several days forming a honey-colored crust. Healing is usually complete within 3 weeks.
B. Immunosuppressed patients, especially HIV infected patients, have more frequent and more severe infections. Contact with ulcerative lesions or with secretions may result in transmission. Asymptomatic viral shedding may also cause infection.
C. Recurrent disease
1. Ninety percent of symptomatic HSV-2 infections and 60% of HSV-1 infections recur within 1 year, but some may have outbreaks as frequently as every 2-3 weeks. The frequency and number of recurrences are highly variable.
2. Recurrent lesions usually arise at the site of the primary infection. Over time, the recurrences become less frequent. Reported precipitating events for recurrent infection include menstruation, stress, sun exposure, cold, and local trauma.

III. Laboratory tests
A. Diagnosis of genital herpes requires the characteristic history and physical appearance of lesions plus the selective use of immunofluorescent assay

or viral culture.

B. Immunofluorescent assays rapidly detects HSV in smears. Viral culture requires 48-96 hours and has an accuracy rate of 85-90%. Serologies are not useful since antibodies become permanently positive after infection.

Treatment of HSV Infections		
Type of infection	**Dosage/regimen**	**Considerations**
Primary infection	**Acyclovir (Zovirax)** 400 mg PO tid x 10 days [Tab 400, 800 mg; cap 200 mg] or **Valacyclovir (Valtrex)** 500 mg PO bid x 10 days or **Famciclovir (Famvir)** 125 mg PO bid x 10 days	Preferred route in immuno-competent patients
	Acyclovir (Zovirax) 5 mg/kg IV q8h over one hour for 5-7 or until clinical resolution	Only for severe symptoms or complications
Recurrent infection Episodic therapy	**Acyclovir (Zovirax)** 400 mg PO tid or 800 mg bid for 5 days or **Valacyclovir (Valtrex)** 500 mg PO bid for 5 days or **Famciclovir (Famvir)** 125 mg PO bid for 5 days	Treatment is most effective when initiated at the earliest sign of recurrence; it is of no benefit if initiated more than 48 hours after symptom onset
Suppressive therapy	**Acyclovir (Zovirax)** 400 mg PO bid	Indicated for patients with frequent and/or severe recurrences (>6 outbreaks/year)

C. Acyclovir (Zovirax) is the drug of choice for the treatment and suppression of genital herpes. It is usually well tolerated, but nausea, vomiting, rash, or headache occur rarely. Topical acyclovir is not effective. Serious or life-threatening HSV infections require intravenous acyclovir.

D. Other antivirals have more convenient bid dosing, but are more expensive than acyclovir and not more effective.
  1. **Valacyclovir (Valtrex)** 500 mg bid x 5 days.
  2. **Famciclovir (Famvir)** 125 mg bid x 5 days.

E. Oral analgesics and sitz baths are useful. The area should be kept clean and dry with corn starch, baby powder, or a hair dryer. Pyridium may be useful for dysuria.

IV. Patient counseling
  A. Patients should be warned about HSV autoinoculation from one body site to another. Infected areas should be patted dry rather than wiped dry. Sunscreen and lip balm are recommended to reduce recurrent disease.
  B. Patients should be advised to abstain from sexual activity while lesions are present. Use of latex condoms is encouraged because of asymptomatic viral shedding.
  C. The risk of neonatal transmission must be explained to the patient.
  D. Recommended testing includes evaluation for gonorrhea, chlamydia, syphilis, genital warts, and human immunodeficiency virus (HIV).

V. Treatment of recurrences
  A. Episodic acyclovir therapy. Early initiation of therapy has been shown to produce a reduction in the duration of symptoms. The patient should keep

a supply of acyclovir and begin treatment at the earliest prodromal symptom.
  B. **Suppressive acyclovir therapy**
    1. Suppressive acyclovir therapy has been shown to reduce the frequency of recurrence by 80% and to prevent recurrence in 30% of patients. Suppressive therapy is recommended when recurrences occur more than 6 times/year.
    2. A suppressive regimen could be used during periods of increased stress or when optimal protection is desired, such as during a vacation or before a wedding.

References: See page 195.

Herpes Zoster

Zoster usually presents as a painful unilateral dermatomal eruption. Zoster results from reactivation of varicella-zoster (chickenpox) virus which has been dormant in the dorsal root ganglia.
  I. **Clinical Evaluation**
    A. Zoster is usually heralded by dermatomal pain, sometimes accompanied by fever. Within a few days, the skin overlying the dermatome reddens and blisters. A few vesicles are usually grouped on one erythematous base, in contrast to the scattered, single vesicles of chickenpox. Several days later the vesicles become pustular and develop crusts, followed by scabs.
    B. Zoster may occur in any dermatome, but the thoracic dermatomes are most often affected. In 90% of patients, pain eventually disappears completely.
    C. The frequency of zoster increases markedly after age 55, but people of any age can be affected. Less than 5% of immunocompetent patients who have one episode of herpes zoster will have another, and the episodes are usually separated by years. HIV-infected patients are more likely to have recurrent herpes zoster infections.
    D. **Laboratory evaluation**
      1. The diagnosis of herpes zoster can be made on clinical grounds without the need for laboratory tests. Viral isolation and culture assays are not useful for varicella-zoster.
      2. An isolated case of zoster in an apparently healthy young or middle-aged adult is probably not an indicator of an underlying immunodeficiency. HIV testing is considered when a patient who engages in high-risk behavior (sexual activities, drug use) develops zoster. Testing for HIV is also indicated when herpes zoster is protracted, recurrent, or involves multiple dermatomes.
    E. **Complications of herpes zoster**
      1. 15% of patients with zoster have involvement of the ophthalmic branch of the trigeminal nerve. Hutchinson's sign, a lesion on the tip of the nose, indicates corneal involvement; however, ophthalmic involvement. Treatment with IV acyclovir and topical agents is required to prevent blindness.
      2. Disseminated herpes zoster is present when 20 or more lesions occur outside of the primary contiguous dermatomes. These patients are at risk for visceral dissemination.
 II. **Therapy for zoster**
    A. Wet dressings or compresses with Burow's solution (Domeboro) will protect sensitive areas. Acetaminophen, nonsteroidal anti-inflammatory drugs, or analgesics with codeine (Vicodin) may be needed.
    B. **Antiviral therapy for zoster**
      1. An antiviral can hasten the resolution of the rash by several days. Relief of acute pain occurs two to three days after an antiviral is initiated. The

duration of pain is reduced by about half. Antiviral therapy is more likely to be of benefit if initiated within 24 hours of rash onset.

2. **Acyclovir (Zovirax)**
   a. 800 mg q4h while awake (5 times a day) for 7 days. [400, 800 mg tab].
   b. Oral acyclovir does not have significant adverse effects; nausea, headaches, diarrhea, and constipation may sometimes occur.
   c. IV acyclovir is reserved for the severely immunosuppressed (bone marrow transplant patients), disseminated infection, or ophthalmic zoster.
   d. The IV dose for zoster is 10 mg/kg, administered over a one-hour, q8h. Nephrotoxicity can usually be avoided if the patient remains well-hydrated. The dosage should be reduced in renal failure.
3. **Famciclovir (Famvir)** is equally effective as acyclovir; it has a more convenient dosing interval; one 500-mg tablet tid for 7 days.
4. **Valacyclovir (Valtrex)**, may be slightly more effective than acyclovir; 1,000 mg tid x 7 days [500 mg].
5. **Foscarnet (Foscavir)** is useful for acyclovir-resistant herpes infections.
6. Ophthalmic distribution zoster is a medical emergency which requires IV acyclovir and topical antivirals.

III. Postherpetic neuralgia
   A. PNH is the most common complication of herpes zoster. It is defined as chronic pain persisting for at least one month after the skin lesions have healed.
   B. The incidence of PHN after an episode of herpes zoster is 5-50%. Those aged 60 and older have a 50% chance of developing PHN. PHN resolves within two months in about half of those affected.
   C. Antivirals, aspirin, and acetaminophen are usually not effective for PHN.
   D. **Topical preparations**
   1. Capsaicin cream OTC (Zostrix, Zostrix-HP) 0.025% tid-qid reduces the pain. Ben-Gay, Flex-all 454 or Aspercreme may offer similar relief.
   2. EMLA topical cream (lidocaine and prilocaine) qid may be useful.
   3. Amitriptyline (Elavil) is often effective; 10-25 mg qhs, increasing in weekly increments of 25 mg as needed.
   4. Gabapentin (Neurontin),   300 mg qd-tid, may be effective. Carbamazepine (Tegretol), 200 mg bid, has also been used.
   5. Transcutaneous electrical nerve stimulation (TENS), lidocaine injections, nerve block injections, permanent nerve blocks with alcohol, and nerve resectioning have been used for recalcitrant cases.

References: See page 195.

Syphilis

Syphilis, an infection caused by *Treponema pallidum*, is usually sexually transmitted and is characterized by episodes of active disease interrupted by periods of latency. About 20,000 cases of primary and secondary syphilis and 32,000 cases of early latent syphilis are reported each year.

I. Clinical evaluation
   A. **Primary syphilis**
   1. The incubation period for syphilis is 10-90 days; 21 days is average.
   2. The lesion begins as a painless, solitary nodule that becomes an indurated ulceration (chancre) with a ham-colored, eroded surface, and a serous discharge found on or near the genitalia. Atypical lesions are frequent and may take the form of small multiple lesions.
   3. The chancre is usually accompanied by painless, enlarged regional lymph nodes. Untreated lesions heal in 1-5 weeks.

    4. The diagnosis is made by the clinical appearance and a positive darkfield examination; the serologic test (VDRL, RPR) is often negative in early disease.

B. Secondary syphilis

    1. Twenty five percent of untreated patients progress to secondary syphilis 2-6 months after exposure. Secondary syphilis lasts for 4-6 weeks.

    2. Bilateral, symmetrical, macular, papular, or papulosquamous skin lesions become widespread. The lesions are non-pruritic and frequently involve the palms, soles, face, trunk and extremities. Condyloma lata consists of rash and moist lesions. Secondary syphilis is highly infectious. Mucous membranes are often involved, appearing as white patches in the mouth, nose, vagina, and rectum.

    3. Generalized nontender lymphadenopathy and patchy alopecia sometimes occur. A small percentage of patients have iritis, hepatitis, meningitis, fever, and headache.

    4. The serologic test (VDRL. RPR) is positive in >99% of cases; the test may be falsely negative because of the prozone phenomenon caused by high antigen titers. Retesting of a diluted blood sample may be positive. No culture test is available.

C. Latent syphilis consists of the interval between secondary syphilis and late syphilis. Patients have no signs or symptoms, only positive serological tests.

D. Late syphilis is characterized by destruction of tissue, organs, and organ systems.

    1. Late benign syphilis. Gummas occur in skin or bone.

    2. Cardiovascular syphilis. Medial necrosis of the aorta may lead to aortic insufficiency or aortic aneurysms.

    3. Neurosyphilis

        a. Spinal fluid shows elevated WBCs, increased total protein, and positive serology.

        b. Pupillary changes are common; the Argyll Robertson pupil accommodates but does not react to light.

        c. Neurosyphilis may cause general paresis or tabes dorsalis--degeneration of the ascending sensory neurons in the posterior columns of the spinal cord.

II. Serology

A. Nontreponemal tests

    1. Complement fixation tests (VDRL or RPR) are used for screening; they become positive 4-6 weeks after infection. The tests start in low titer and, over several weeks, may reach 1:32 or higher. After adequate treatment of primary syphilis, the titer falls becomes nonreactive within 9-18 months.

    2. False positive tests occur in hepatitis, mononucleosis, viral pneumonia, malaria, varicella, autoimmune diseases, diseases associated with increased globulins, narcotic addicts, leprosy, and old age.

B. Treponemal tests

    1. Treponemal tests include the FTA-ABS test, TPI test, and microhemagglutination assay for T. pallidum (MHA-TP). A treponemal test should be used to confirm a positive VDRL or RPR.

    2. Treponemal tests are specific to treponema antibodies and will remain positive after treatment. All patients with syphilis should be tested for HIV.

III. Treatment of primary or secondary syphilis

A. Primary or secondary syphilis. Benzathine penicillin G, 2.4 million units IM in a single dose.

B. Patients who have syphilis and who also have symptoms or signs suggesting neurologic disease (meningitis) or ophthalmic disease (uveitis) should be fully evaluated for neurosyphilis and syphilitic eye disease (CSF analysis and ocular slit-lamp examination).

    C. **Penicillin allergic patients.** Doxycycline 100 mg PO 2 times a day for 2 weeks.

    D. **Follow-up and retreatment**
       1. Early syphilis--repeat VDRL at 3, 6, and 12 months to ensure that titers are declining.
       2. Syphilis >1 year--also repeat VDRL at 24 months.
       3. Neurosyphilis-- also repeat VDRL for 3 years.
       4. **Indications for retreatment**
         a. Clinical signs or symptoms persist or recur.
         b. 4-fold increase in the titer of a nontreponemal test (VDRL).
         c. Failure of an initially high titer nontreponemal test (VDRL) to show a 4-fold decrease within a year.
       5. Sex partners should be evaluated and treated.

IV. Treatment of latent syphilis
    A. Patients who have latent syphilis who have acquired syphilis within the preceding year are classified as having early latent syphilis. Latent syphilis of unknown duration should be managed as late latent syphilis.
    B. **Treatment of early latent syphilis.** Benzathine penicillin G, 2.4 million units IM in a single dose.
    C. **Treatment of late latent syphilis or latent syphilis of unknown duration** Benzathine penicillin G 2.4 million units IM each week x 3 weeks.
    D. All patients should be evaluated clinically for evidence of late syphilis (aortitis, neurosyphilis, gumma, iritis).
    E. **Indications for CSF examination before treatment**
       1. Neurologic or ophthalmic signs or symptoms
       2. Other evidence of active syphilis (aortitis, gumma, iritis)
       3. Treatment failure
       4. HIV infection
       5. Serum nontreponemal titer >1:32, unless duration of infection is known to be <1 year
       6. Nonpenicillin therapy planned, unless duration of infection is known to be <1 year.
    F. **CSF examination** includes cell count, protein, and CSF-VDRL. If a CSF examination is performed and the results are abnormal, the patient should be treated for neurosyphilis.

V. Treatment of late syphilis
    A. Benzathine penicillin G 2.4 million units IM weekly x 3 weeks. Penicillin allergic patients are treated with doxycycline 100 mg PO bid x 4 weeks.
    B. Patients with late syphilis should undergo CSF examination before therapy.

VI. Treatment of neurosyphilis
    A. Central nervous system disease can occur during any stage of syphilis. Clinical evidence of neurologic involvement (eg, ophthalmic or auditory symptoms, cranial nerve palsies) warrants a CSF examination. Patients with CSF abnormalities should have follow-up CSF examinations to assess response to treatment.
    B. **Treatment of neurosyphilis.** Penicillin G 2-4 million units IV q4h for 10-14 days. Alternatively, penicillin G procaine 2.4 million units IM daily plus probenecid 500 mg PO qid, both for 10-14 days can be used.
    C. **Follow-up.** If CSF pleocytosis was present initially, CSF examination should be repeated every 6 months until the cell count is normal. Follow-up CSF examinations also may be used to evaluate changes in the VDRL-CSF or CSF protein in response to therapy.

References: See page 195.

Tuberculosis

One-third of the world population is infected with tuberculosis. The tuberculosis case rate in the United States is 9.4 cases per 100,000 population.

I. **Pathophysiology**

A. In most individuals infected with mycobacterium tuberculosis (by respiratory aerosols), the primary pulmonary infection occurs early in life, and the organism is contained by host defenses. The primary infection usually resembles pneumonia or bronchitis, and the infection usually resolves without treatment.

B. After the immune system limits spread of the bacilli during the primary infection, patients are typically asymptomatic, although the organisms may remain viable and dormant for many years. In these individuals, the only indication of primary infection is conversion to a positive reaction to the purified protein derivative (PPD) skin test. Acid-fast bacilli are not present in the sputum.

C. Later in life, the organism may cause reactivation disease, usually pulmonary, but it may affect the genitourinary system, bones, joints, meninges, brain, peritoneum, and pericardium. Reactivation of tuberculosis is the most common form of clinically apparent disease. Immunocompetent individuals with tuberculosis infection have a 10% chance of developing reactivation disease during their lifetimes. In HIV positive patients, the risk of acquiring active TB is 10% per year.

II. **Diagnosis of active pulmonary tuberculosis**

A. Chronic cough with scant sputum production and blood streaking of sputum are the most common symptoms of pulmonary disease. Pulmonary tuberculosis should be considered in any patient with the following characteristics:

1. cough for more than 3 weeks
2. night sweats
3. bloody sputum or hemoptysis
4. weight loss
5. fever
6. anorexia
7. history of exposure to tuberculosis, institutionalization, HIV infection, or a positive PPD test.

B. Diagnosis of active pulmonary tuberculosis rests upon sputum examination for acid fast bacilli and subsequent culture and sensitivities. This process requires 4-6 weeks for identification and another 4-6 weeks for sensitivity testing. Smears and cultures should be performed on three different days in patients at high risk for infection.

C. DNA probes that use polymerase chain reactions (PCR) are available for more rapid identification of tuberculosis. They are useful for making an early diagnosis of Tb while awaiting culture results.

D. **Chest radiographs**

1. **Reactivation pulmonary tuberculosis** is characterized by infiltrates in the apical and posterior segments of the upper lobes or in the superior segments of the lower lobes.
2. **Cavitation** is frequently present in regions of substantial infiltration. Lordotic views, taken in an anterior-posterior fashion with the patient leaning backward, allow better visualization of the lung apices.

E. **Skin testing for tuberculosis**

1. The purified protein derivative (PPD) test is a reliable method of recognizing prior infection, however, it is neither sensitive nor specific. It is useful in detecting patients who are harboring latent tuberculosis who may need "prophylactic" therapy. The test is read at 48-72 hrs.
2. False-positive reactions are possible as a result of exposure to non-pathological mycobacterial disease (eg, M. avium complex). False-

negative reactions are seen with advancing age and immunosuppression. Twenty five percent of all individuals with active tuberculosis have a negative skin test. A history of vaccination with bacille Calmette-Guerin (BCG) should be ignored when interpreting the results of tuberculin skin testing because skin test reactivity from the vaccine wanes after 2 years.

Interpretation of PPD Results

1. **Induration ≥5 mm is considered positive in:**
   - HIV-positive individuals
   - persons with recent close contact with individual with active tuberculosis
   - persons with chest x-ray consistent with healed tuberculosis

2. **Induration ≥10 mm is considered positive in:**
   High-Risk Groups
   - intravenous drug users who are HIV negative
   - patients with chronic illness at risk for reactivation (silicosis, chronic renal failure, diabetes mellitus, chronic steroid use, hematologic disorders, malignancy)
   - children younger than 4 years of age
   High-Prevalence Groups
   - immigrants from endemic regions (Asia, Africa, Latin America, Caribbean)
   - residents of long-term care facilities (nursing homes, prisons)
   - persons from medically underserved, low-income populations

3. **Induration ≥15 mm is considered positive in all persons.**

4. **Recent conversion criteria:**
   - increase ≥10 mm within two years in individuals younger than 35 years of age
   - increase ≥15 mm within two years in individuals 35 years of age or older

5. **Interpretation of PPD Testing in health care workers:**
   - follow guidelines 1-3
   - facilities with a high prevalence of tuberculosis patients may consider induration 10 mm in individuals without other risk factors as a positive reaction
   - recent conversion is an increase in induration of 10 mm in a two-year period in high-prevalence facilities, 15 mm in low-prevalence facilities

---

    F. Tuberculosis is often the initial manifestation of HIV infection; therefore, serologic testing for HIV is recommended in all tuberculosis patients.

III. **Chemoprophylaxis for patients with a positive PPD**
    A. Chemoprophylaxis with isoniazid (INH) greatly decreases the likelihood of progression of latent tuberculous infection to active disease. Before administration of chemoprophylaxis, active tuberculosis must be excluded clinically and by chest x-ray.

Preventive Therapy Considerations

General Population
- Individuals <35 years of age with positive reaction to PPD (including children)
- HIV-positive patients with positive PPD reactions
- Anergic individuals with recent known contact to person(s) with active tuberculosis
- Children with known TB exposure, even if PPD negative

Health Care Workers
(in addition to above recommendations)
- Recent PPD conversion
- Close contact of individual with active tuberculosis
- HIV-positive, regardless of PPD reaction
- Intravenous drug users
- Medical condition that increases risk of progression to active disease

Preventative Therapy Recommendations

Isoniazid
   300 mg po daily in adults
   10 mg/kg po daily in children

Duration
   6-12 months in otherwise healthy adults
   9 months in children
   12 months in HIV-positive individuals

If exposure to INH resistant organisms has been documented, prophylaxis should be attempted with rifampin and ethambutol for 12 months.

IV. Treatment of active tuberculosis
   A. Suspected TB should be treated empirically with a 4 drug combination. The four-drug regimen consists of isoniazid, rifampin, pyrazinamide, and ethambutol. Patients should be treated for 8 weeks with the four-drug regimen, followed by 16 weeks of INH and rifampin daily or 2-3 times weekly. HIV-positive patients should be treated for a total of 9 months and at least 6 months following culture conversion to negative.
   B. If multi-drug resistant TB (resistant to both INH and RIF) is encountered, therapy should be more prolonged and guided by antibiotic sensitivities. Directly observed therapy, on a twice per week basis, should be instituted when compliance is questioned.

Dosage Recommendations for Treatment of Tuberculosis

Drug	Daily Dose	Two Times/week Dose	Three Times/week Dose
Isoniazid (INH)	5 mg/kg, max 300 mg	15 mg/kg, max 900 mg	15 mg/kg, max 900 mg

Rifampin (RIF)	10 mg/kg, max 600 mg	10 mg/kg, max 600 mg	10 mg/kg, max 600 mg
Pyrazinamide (PZA)	15-30 mg/kg, max 2 g	50-70 mg/kg, max 4 g	50-70 mg/kg, max 3 g
Ethambutol (EMB)	5-25 mg/kg, max 2.5 g	50 mg/kg, max 2.5 g	25-30 mg/kg, max 2.5 g
Streptomycin (SM)	15 mg/kg, max 1 g	25-30 mg/kg, max 1.5 g	25-30 mg/kg, max 1 g

Initial Treatment of Tuberculosis

HIV Negative

INH + RIF + PZA + (EMB) daily for eight weeks followed by INH + RIF daily or 2-3 times weekly for 16 weeks.
Regimen may be tailored following results of susceptibility testing.

HIV Positive

Continue above regimen for a total of nine months and at least six months following culture conversion to negative.

C. Symptoms should improve within 4 weeks, and sputum cultures should become negative within 3 months in patients receiving effective antituberculosis therapy.
D. Sputum cultures should be obtained monthly until they are negative, and cultures should be obtained after completion of therapy. A chest x-ray should be obtained after 2-3 months and after completion of treatment to assess efficacy.

References: See page 195.

Tetanus Prophylaxis

History of Two Primary Immunizations:
    Low risk wound - Tetanus toxoid 0.5 mL IM.
    Tetanus prone - Tetanus toxoid 0.5 mL IM + Tetanus immunoglobulin (TIG) 250-500 U IM.
Three Primary and 10 yrs since last Booster:
    Low risk wound - Tetanus toxoid, 0.5 mL IM.
    Tetanus prone - Tetanus toxoid, 0.5 mL IM.
Three Primary and 5-10 yrs since last Booster:
    Low risk wound - None
    Tetanus prone - Tetanus toxoid, 0.5 mL IM.
Three Primary and ≤5 yrs since last Booster:
    Low risk wound - None
    Tetanus prone - None

Infectious Conjunctivitis

Infectious conjunctivitis is one of the most common causes of red eye. Infectious conjunctivitis is commonly caused by bacterial or viral infection. The clinical term "red eye" is applied to a variety of infectious or inflammatory diseases of the eye. Conjunctivitis is most frequently caused by a bacterial or viral infection. Sexually transmitted diseases such as chlamydial infection and gonorrhea are less common causes of conjunctivitis. Ocular allergy is a major cause of chronic conjunctivitis.

I. **Clinical evaluation of conjunctivitis**
   A. The history should establish whether the condition is acute, subacute, chronic or recurrent, and whether it is unilateral or bilateral.
   B. **Discharge**
      1. **Serous discharge (watery)** is most commonly associated with viral or allergic ocular conditions.
      2. **Mucoid discharge (stringy or ropy)** is highly characteristic of allergy or dry eyes.
      3. **Mucopurulent or purulent discharge,** often associated with morning crusting and difficulty opening the eyelids, strongly suggests a bacterial infection. The possibility of *Neisseria gonorrhoeae* infection should be considered when the discharge is copiously purulent.

Differential Diagnosis of Red Eye	

Conjunctivitis
  Infectious
    Viral
    Bacterial (eg, staphylococcus,
    Chlamydia)
  Noninfectious
    Allergic conjunctivitis
    Dry eye
    Toxic or chemical reaction
    Contact lens use
    Foreign body
    Factitious conjunctivitis
	Keratitis
	    Infectious. Bacterial, viral, fungal
	    Noninfectious. Recurrent epithelial
	    erosion, foreign body
	Uveitis
	Episcleritis/scleritis
	Acute glaucoma
	Eyelid abnormalities
	Orbital disorders
	    Preseptal and orbital cellulitis
	    Idiopathic orbital inflammation
	    (pseudotumor)

   C. **Itching** is highly suggestive of allergic conjunctivitis. A history of recurrent itching or a personal or family history of hay fever, allergic rhinitis, asthma or atopic dermatitis is also consistent with ocular allergy.
   D. **Unilateral or bilateral conjunctivitis**. Bilateral conjunctivitis suggests allergic conjunctivitis. Unilateral conjunctivitis is associated with infections caused by viruses and bacteria.
   E. **Pain, photophobia and blurred vision.** Pain and photophobia do not usually occur with conjunctivitis, and these findings suggest an ocular or orbital disease processes, including uveitis, keratitis, acute glaucoma or orbital cellulitis. Blurred vision is not characteristic of conjunctivitis. This finding is indicative of corneal or intraocular pathology.
   F. **Recent contact with an individual with an upper respiratory tract infection** suggests adenoviral conjunctivitis. Chlamydial or gonococcal infection may be suggested by the patient's sexual history, including a history of urethral discharge.

II. **Examination of the eye**
   A. Visual acuity should be tested before the examination. Regional lymphadenopathy should be sought and the face and eyelids examined. Viral or chlamydial inclusion conjunctivitis typically presents with a tender, preauricular or submandibular lymph node. Palpable adenopathy is rare

in acute bacterial conjunctivitis. Herpes labialis or a dermatomal vesicular eruption (suggestive of shingles) is indicative of a herpetic conjunctivitis.

B. Purulent discharge suggests a bacterial infection. Stringy mucoid discharge suggests allergy. Clear watery discharge suggests viral infection.

Discharge Associated with Conjunctivitis				
Etiology	Serous	Mucoid	Mucopuru-lent	Purulent
Viral	+	-	-	-
Bacterial	-	-	+	+
Allergic	+	+	-	-
Chlamydial	-	+	+	-

III. **Cultures and Gram stain** usually are not required in patients with mild conjunctivitis of suspected viral, bacterial or allergic origin. However, bacterial cultures should be obtained in patients who have severe conjunctivitis.

IV. **Treatment of bacterial conjunctivitis**

  A. Acute bacterial conjunctivitis typically presents with burning, irritation, tearing and a mucopurulent or purulent discharge. The three most common pathogens in bacterial conjunctivitis are *Streptococcus pneumoniae, Haemophilus influenzae* and *Staphylococcus aureus.*

  B. **Topical broad-spectrum antibiotics** such as erythromycin ointment and bacitracin-polymyxin B ointment as well as combination solutions such as trimethoprim-polymyxin B provide excellent coverage for most conjunctival pathogens. Ointments are better tolerated by young children. Solutions are preferred by adults.

   1. **Erythromycin ophthalmic ointment,** apply to affected eye(s) q3-4h.
   2. **Bacitracin-polymyxin B (Polysporin)** ophthalmic ointment or solution, apply to affected eye(s) q3-4h.
   3. **Trimethoprim-polymyxin B (Polytrim)**, ointment or solution, apply to affected eye(s) q3-4h.

  C. **Conjunctivitis due to H. influenzae, N. gonorrhoeae, and N. meningitidis** requires systemic antibiotic therapy in addition to topical treatment. Gonococcal conjunctivitis may be treated with ceftriaxone (Rocephin) 1 g IM and topical erythromycin.

  D. **Chlamydial conjunctivitis** can be present in newborns, in sexually active teenagers and in adults. Diagnosis is by antibody staining of ocular samples. Treatment includes oral tetracycline, doxycycline (Vibramycin) or erythromycin for two weeks.

V. **Viral conjunctivitis**

  A. Adenovirus is the most common cause of viral conjunctivitis. Viral conjunctivitis often occurs in epidemics, typically presenting with an acutely red eye, watery discharge, conjunctival swelling, a tender preauricular node, photophobia and a foreign-body sensation. Some patients have an associated upper respiratory tract infection.

  B. **Treatment** consists of cold compresses and topical vasoconstrictors (Vasocon-A, Naphcon-A). Patients should avoid direct contact with other persons for at least one week after the onset of symptoms.

  C. **Ocular herpes simplex** and herpes zoster is managed with topical agents, including trifluridine (Viroptic) and systemic acyclovir, famciclovir or valacyclovir.

References: See page 195.

Gastrointestinal Disorders

Gastroesophageal Reflux Disease

One-third of the population experiences symptoms of heartburn at least monthly. The severity of gastroesophageal reflux disease (GERD) ranges from occasional mild symptoms to severe, erosive esophagitis with complications of ulcer, stricture, and hemorrhage.

I. Clinical evaluation of gastroesophageal reflux disease
   A. The most common symptom of GERD is heartburn, a burning sensation in the epigastric or retrosternal area, often occurring postprandially. Regurgitation, dysphagia, and belching may also occur.
   B. Hoarseness, nocturnal cough, and wheezing may be caused by chronic reflux, and asthma may be exacerbated by GERD.
   C. Chronic reflux is associated with Barrett's esophagus (columnar metaplasia of esophageal mucosa). This complication may predispose to esophageal adenocarcinoma.
   D. GERD is caused by decreased lower esophageal sphincter (LES) pressure. Sphincter tone can be impaired by consumption of fatty foods and anticholinergic medications.

II. Therapeutic approach to gastroesophageal reflux disease
   A. Empiric therapy. When classic symptoms (heartburn) are present, a presumptive diagnosis of GERD may be made and treatment initiated.
   B. Non-pharmacologic therapy for gastroesophageal reflux disease
      1. Initial therapy consists of diet and lifestyle modifications and use of antacids as needed. Lifestyle modifications include weight loss, reduced dietary fat, limitation of caffeine, chocolate and peppermint. Meals should be smaller and more frequent, and smoking and alcohol should be limited.
      2. Elevation of the head of the bed and avoidance of recumbency for three hours after a meal is recommended.
      3. The patient's medications should be reviewed for drugs that exacerbate GERD, including alpha-adrenergic blockers, anticholinergics, benzodiazepines, beta-adrenergic agonists, calcium channel blockers, narcotics, nitrates, progestins, and transdermal nicotine.
   C. Acid-suppressive treatment
      1. Patients who continue to have symptoms should be offered an acid-suppressive treatment
      2. The four available H_2-blockers are equally safe and effective. A twice-daily schedule should be used to provide 24-hour acid control.

Pharmacologic Treatment of Gastroesophageal Reflux Disease		
Agent	Dosage	
Histamine-2 blockers: Inhibit gastric acid secretion		
Ranitidine (Zantac) Famotidine (Pepcid) Nizatidine (Axid) Cimetidine (Tagamet)	150-300 mg bid 20-40 mg bid 150-300 mg bid 400-800 mg bid	Cimetidine may cause impotence and gynecomastia; many drug interactions

Agent	Dosage	
Prokinetic drugs: Increase lower esophageal sphincter pressure, increase peristalsis		
Cisapride (Propulsid)	Up to 20 mg qid [10 mg]	Mild diarrhea
Proton-pump inhibitors: Inhibit gastric acid secretion		
Omeprazole (Prilosec) Lansoprazole (Prevacid)	20 mg qd or bid 30 mg qd	8 weeks of treatment

- D. **Promotility drugs–cisapride (Propulsid)**.
  1. Cisapride increases lower esophageal sphincter pressure and promotes peristalsis. Some studies have shown cisapride to have efficacy equal to that of H2 receptor antagonists.
  2. Cisapride may also be its used in combination with acid suppression therapy. Cisapride works synergistically with H2 receptor antagonists to promote esophageal healing and reduce symptoms.
  3. Cisapride is well tolerated, and side effects are limited to mild gastrointestinal symptoms, most notably diarrhea.
- E. **Persistent symptoms**
  1. For patients with persistent symptoms following 6 weeks of H2 blocker therapy, or for patients initially presenting with dysphagia, hemorrhage, or severe disease, further diagnostic evaluation is necessary, which may include an upper GI series, esophageal endoscopy, biopsy, or pH monitoring.
  2. Treatment options for persistent symptoms include combination of an H_2-blocker with a promotility drug, or switching to omeprazole (Prilosec).
  3. **Omeprazole (Prilosec)**
     - a. Omeprazole is more effective than H_2-blockers in symptom relief (83%) and in healing of esophagitis (78%).
     - b. The majority of patients will respond to omeprazole 20 mg qd. Some patients may require 20 mg bid is rarely required.
  4. **Lansoprazole (Prevacid)** appears to be similarly effective to omeprazole at a dosage of 30 mg qd.
  5. **Anti-reflux surgery**
     - a. Surgery is recommended only for patients who are resistant to or intolerant of medical therapy or who have complications of GERD (eg, recurrent aspiration esophageal stricture formation).
     - b. Antireflux surgery has shown disappointing long-term results, and is indicated only on rare occasions.
     - c. **Nissen fundoplication** is the most commonly used operation. The fundus is completely wrapped around the esophagus, and the hiatus is closed. The procedure is usually done laparoscopically.

References: See page 195.

Peptic Ulcer Disease

Peptic ulcer disease is diagnosed in 500,000 patients each year in the United States.

I. **Pathophysiology**

    A. Helicobacter pylori (HP), a spiral-shaped, flagellated organism, is the most frequent cause of peptic ulcer disease (PUD). Nonsteroidal anti-inflammatory drugs (NSAIDs) and pathologically high acid-secreting states (Zollinger-Ellison syndrome) are less common causes. More than 90% of ulcers are associated with H. pylori. Eradication of the organism cures and prevents relapses of gastroduodenal ulcers.

    B. **Complications of peptic ulcer disease** include bleeding, duodenal or gastric perforation, and gastric outlet obstruction (due to inflammation or strictures).

II. **Clinical evaluation**

    A. **Symptoms of PUD** include recurrent upper abdominal pain and discomfort. The pain of duodenal ulceration is often relieved by food and antacids and worsened when the stomach is empty (eg, at nighttime). In gastric ulceration, the pain may be exacerbated by eating.

    B. **Nausea and vomiting** are common in PUD. Hematemesis ("coffee ground" emesis) or melena (black tarry stools) are indicative of bleeding.

    C. **Physical examination.** Tenderness to deep palpation is often present in the epigastrium, and the stool is often guaiac-positive.

III. **Laboratory detection of Helicobacter pylori infection**

    A. **Non-endoscopic tests for H pylori infection**

        1. For the initial diagnosis, serologic testing is recommended for most patients with uncomplicated PUD. Patients over the age of 50 and patients with gastrointestinal bleeding, weight loss, vomiting or severe pain, or patients who do not respond to therapy within two weeks should be evaluated with endoscopy.

        2. **Serologic tests** have a sensitivity of 80-95 % and specificity is 80-96%. Serology is relatively inexpensive. H pylori antibodies persist for several years after H. pylori eradication. Therefore, serology is useful in the initial diagnosis of H. priori infection, but it is not useful as a test of cure following antibiotic treatment.

        3. **Breath tests using C-13-labeled urea** are more expensive than serology but have a sensitivity of >95% and a specificity >95%. The urea breath test can be used for initial diagnosis and as a test of cure.

    B. **Endoscopic testing for H pylori infection** is the most sensitive method of detecting gastric and duodenal ulceration.

IV. **Treatment of peptic ulcer disease and eradication of H pylori infection**

    A. **Antibiotic regimens for H. pylori infection**

        1. **Dual therapy** uses omeprazole (a proton pump inhibitor) in combination with metronidazole (Flagyl) and clarithromycin (Biaxin). This regimen is >90% effective in H. pylori eradication and is simpler than Triple Therapy.

        2. **Triple therapy** uses Pepto Bismol in combination with metronidazole and either tetracycline or amoxicillin. This regimen is effective in eradicating H. pylori infection in >90%. It is inexpensive, but has the disadvantage of being complicated.

Antibiotic Regimens for H Pylori Infection	
Dual Therapy	**Triple Therapy**
Omeprazole (Prilosec) 20 mg bid. **Metronidazole (Flagyl)** 500 mg bid. **Clarithromycin (Biaxin)** 250 mg bid. 10 days of therapy is 95% effective. If active ulcer, continue omeprazole, 20 mg qd, for an additional 2-3 weeks.	**Pepto-Bismol** 2 tablets qid. **Metronidazole** 250 mg qid. **Tetracycline or Amoxicillin** 500 mg qid. 14 days of therapy is 95% effective. If active ulcer, treat with H2-blocker for 4-6 weeks.

    B. Follow-up after treatment of H pylori. Patients with uncomplicated peptic ulcer disease treated for H pylori infection do not require a "test of cure" to confirm eradication of H. pylori. However, if their symptoms return, further evaluation for recurrent or persistent H. pylori infection is required.

    C. Treatment of NSAID-related ulcers
        1. When the ulcer is caused by NSAID use, healing of the ulcer is greatly facilitated by discontinuing the NSAID. Acid antisecretory therapy with an H2-blocker or proton pump inhibitor speeds ulcer healing.
        2. Proton pump inhibitors are more effective in inhibiting gastric acid production and are often used to heal ulcers in patients who require continuing NSAID treatment.
        3. If serologic or endoscopic testing for H pylori is positive, antibiotic treatment is necessary.

    D. Acute H$_2$-blocker therapy
        1. **Ranitidine (Zantac)**, 150 mg bid or 300 mg qhs.
        2. **Famotidine (Pepcid)**, 20 mg bid or 40 mg qhs.
        3. **Nizatidine (Axid Pulvules)**, 150 mg bid or 300 mg qhs.
        4. **Cimetidine (Tagamet)**, 400 mg bid or 800 mg qhs.

    E. Proton pump inhibitors
        1. **Omeprazole (Prilosec)**, 20 mg qd.
        2. **Lansoprazole (Prevacid)**, 15 mg before breakfast qd.

V. Surgical treatment of peptic ulcer disease
    A. Indications for surgery. Exsanguinating hemorrhage, >5 units transfusion in 24-hours, rebleeding during same hospitalization, intractability, perforation, gastric outlet obstruction, endoscopic signs predictive of rebleeding.
    B. Unstable patients should receive a truncal vagotomy, oversewing of bleeding ulcer bed, and pyloroplasty.

References: See page 195.

Constipation

Constipation affects about 2% of the population, occurring more frequently in persons older than 65.
I. Clinical evaluation
    A. Diagnostic criteria for constipation (2 or more of the following):
        1. Fewer than 3 bowel movements/week.
        2. Excessive straining during bowel movements.
        3. A feeling of incomplete evacuation after bowel movements.

    4. Passage of hard or pellet-like stools.
- **B. Clinical evaluation**
  1. The time of onset of constipation, stool frequency and consistency, the degree of straining, a sensation of complete or incomplete evacuation should be determined.
  2. Chronic suppression of the urge to defecate contributes to constipation. Determine the amount of fiber and fluid consumed. Obstetric, surgical and drug histories, history of back trauma or neurologic problems should be assessed.
- **C. Physical examination**
  1. A palpable colon with stool in the left lower quadrant may be detected, although the examination is often normal. Gastrointestinal masses should be sought. Perianal inspection may reveal skin excoriation, skin tags, anal fissures, anal fistula, or hemorrhoids.
  2. Rectal examination may reveal a mass or stool. Resting and squeeze sphincter tone should be assessed. When the patient is asked to bear down as if to defecate, relaxation of anal tone and perineal descent should be palpable. The absence of anal relaxation or inadequate perineal descent, raises the suspicion of obstructive defecation.
- **D. Laboratory evaluation.** A complete blood cell count, glucose, calcium, phosphate, thyroid function test, calcium, stool examination for ova and parasites, occult blood, and flexible sigmoidoscopy may be indicated to exclude organic causes.
- **E. Secondary causes of constipation**
  1. Fissure in ano, hemorrhoids, fistulas, ischiorectal abscess, colonic neoplasms, hypothyroidism, hypercalcemia, diabetes, Hirschsprung's disease, Parkinson's disease, multiple sclerosis, or cerebrovascular disease may cause constipation.
  2. **Inadequate fiber** intake commonly causes constipation.
  3. **Drugs** that cause constipation include opiate analgesics, aluminum-containing antacids, iron and calcium supplements, antidiarrheals, antihistamines, antidepressants, antiparkinson agents, and calcium channel blockers.
  4. If secondary causes have been excluded, the most likely cause is idiopathic constipation related to a disorder of colorectal motility.

II. Empiric management of constipation
- **A. Behavioral modification.** The patient should be encouraged to heed the urge to defecate and not suppress it. Patients should establish a regular pattern of moving their bowels at the same time every day, usually in the morning, after breakfast. Daily exercise is advised.
- **B. Fiber.** The patient should be placed on a diet of 20-30 g of dietary fiber per day. Fiber must be taken with ample fluids, otherwise constipation may worsen.
- **C.** Laxatives and nonessential drugs should be discontinued.

Fiber Preparations		
Preparation	**Recommended Dose**	**Doses/Day**
Powder		
Metamucil (regular)	1 tsp	1-3
Metamucil (orange flavor or sugar-free)	1 tsp	1-3
Citrucel (orange flavor or sugar-free)	1 tbsp	1-3
Fiberall Natural Flavor	1 tsp	1-3

Preparation	Recommended Dose	Doses/Day
Wafers Metamucil	2	1-3
Tablets Fiberall	1	1-2
Chewable FiberCon	2	1-4

III. Secondary evaluation
   A. If dietary measures are unsuccessful, a secondary evaluation should be undertaken.
   B. **Colonoscopy or barium enema** is necessary to rule out an organic lesion.
   C. **Assessment of colonic transit time**
      1. **The Sitzmarks test** consists of administering a Sitzmarks capsule, containing 24 radiopaque markers. A flat-plate film of the abdomen is obtained 5 days after administration.
      2. The presence of five or more markers spread out in the colon, suggests slow transit of stool through the colon. If markers are closely clustered in the rectosigmoid segment, this indicates obstructive defecation.
   D. **Evaluation of obstructive defecation**
      1. **Anorectal manometry.** A pressure probe is placed in the rectum and anus to assesses the pressure activity.
      2. **Defecography.** Barium is placed in the rectum and the patient bears down during videofluoroscopic imaging.
      3. **Electromyograph.** An electrode is placed in the external anal sphincter and myoelectrical activity is measured.
      4. **Simulated defecation.** A silicone-filled artificial stool is placed in the rectum. Difficulty in expelling the artificial stool indicates obstructive defecation.
IV. Treatment of refractory constipation
   A. **Saline cathartics**, such as magnesium-containing compounds and the phosphate enemas, work by an osmotic effect. Magnesium or phosphate overload may occur in renal insufficiency. Long-term use is not recommended. **Magnesium hydroxide** (1-2 tbsp qd-bid) is most commonly used. In refractory cases, a half to 1 glassful of **magnesium citrate** is effective.
   B. **Lactulose** is a hyperosmotic non-absorbable sugar that is often used for long-term management. Its advantages are nonsystemic absorption, minimal toxicity, and safety for prolonged use; 30 mL PO qd-bid. Sorbitol is significantly less expensive than lactulose; the 70% solution is taken as 30 mL qd-bid.
   C. **Lavage solutions (CoLyte, GoLYTELY)** are used for refractory constipation. These agents contain a balanced electrolyte solution. A gallon can be administered in 4 hours to relieve an impaction. Eight to16 oz a day can be prescribed to prevent recurrence.
   D. **Prokinetic agents** promote peristalsis in the colon. **Cisapride (Propulsid)** increases the frequency of bowel movements in chronically constipated patients at a dose of 10-20 mg qid [10 mg].
   E. **Combination therapy** with an osmotic agent combined with a lavage solution and a prokinetic agent may be used for refractory constipation.
   F. **Enemas** may relieve severe constipation. Low-volume tap water enemas or sodium phosphate (Fleet) enemas can be given once a week to help initiate a bowel movement.
   G. **Stool impaction.** A combination of suppositories (glycerin or bisacodyl)

and enemas (phosphate) will soften the stool. Digital disimpaction may be necessary should these measures fail.

    H. **Surgery.** When the above measures are not effective, surgery may be considered as a last resort. Surgical options include colectomy and ileostomy or an ileoanal pouch.

References: See page 195.

Acute Diarrhea

Acute diarrhea is defined as diarrheal disease of rapid onset, often with nausea, vomiting, fever, or abdominal pain. Most episodes of acute gastroenteritis will resolve within 3 to 7 days.

I. Clinical evaluation of acute diarrhea
    A. The nature of onset, duration, frequency, and timing of the diarrheal episodes should be assessed. The appearance of the stool, buoyancy, presence of blood or mucus, vomiting, or pain should be determined.
    B. Contact with a potential source of infectious diarrhea should be sought.
    C. **Drugs that may cause diarrhea** include laxatives, magnesium-containing compounds, sulfa-drugs, antibiotics.

II. Physical examination
    A. **Assessment of volume status.** Dehydration is suggested by dry mucous membranes, orthostatic hypotension, tachycardia, mental status changes, and acute weight loss.
    B. **Abdominal tenderness**, mild distention and hyperactive bowel sounds are common in acute infectious diarrhea. The presence of peritoneal signs or rigidity suggests toxic megacolon or perforation, requiring radiologic examination of the abdomen.
    C. **Evidence of systemic atherosclerosis** suggests ischemia. Lower extremity edema suggests malabsorption or protein loss.

III. Acute infectious diarrhea
    A. **Infectious diarrhea** is usually classified as noninflammatory or inflammatory, depending on whether the infectious organism has invaded the intestinal mucosa.
    B. **Noninflammatory** infectious diarrhea is caused by organisms that produce a toxin (enterotoxigenic E coli strains, Vibrio cholerae). Noninflammatory, infectious diarrhea is usually self-limiting and lasts less than 3 days.
    C. **Blood or mucus** in the stool suggests inflammatory disease, usually caused by bacterial invasion of the mucosa (enteroinvasive E coli, Shigella, Salmonella, Campylobacter). Patients usually have a septic appearance and fever; some have abdominal rigidity and severe abdominal pain.
    D. **Vomiting out of proportion to diarrhea** is usually related to a neuroenterotoxin-mediated food poisoning from Staphylococcus aureus or Bacillus cereus, or from an enteric virus, such as rotavirus (in an infant), or a small round virus, such as Norwalk virus (in older children or adults). The incubation period for neuroenterotoxin food poisoning is less than 4 hours, while that of a viral agent is more than 8 hours.
    E. **Traveler's diarrhea** is a common acute diarrhea. Three or four unformed stools are passed/24 hours, usually starting on the third day of travel and lasting 2-3 days. Anorexia, nausea, vomiting, abdominal cramps, abdominal bloating, and flatulence may also be present.
    F. Antibiotic-related diarrhea
        1. Antibiotic-related diarrhea ranges from mild illness to life-threatening pseudomembranous colitis. Overgrowth of Clostridium difficile causes pseudomembranous colitis. Amoxicillin, cephalosporins and clindamycin have been implicated most often, but any antibiotic can be the cause.
        2. Patients with pseudomembranous colitis have high fever, cramping,

leukocytosis, and severe, watery diarrhea.

3. Latex agglutination testing for C difficile toxin can provide results in 30 minutes.

4. **Enterotoxigenic E coli**
   a. The enterotoxigenic E coli include the E coli serotype 0157:H7. Grossly bloody diarrhea is most often caused by E. coli 0157:H7, causing 8% of grossly bloody stools.
   b. Enterotoxigenic E coli can cause hemolytic uremic syndrome, thrombotic thrombocytopenic purpura, intestinal perforation, sepsis, and rectal prolapse.

IV. **Diagnostic approach to acute infectious diarrhea**
   A. An attempt should be made to obtain a pathologic diagnosis in patients who give a history of recent ingestion of seafood (Vibrio parahaemolyticus), travel or camping, antibiotic use, homosexual activity, or who complain of fever and abdominal pain.
   B. Blood or mucus in the stools indicates the presence of Shigella, Salmonella, Campylobacter jejuni, enteroinvasive E. coli, C. difficile, or, less likely, Yersinia enterocolitica.
   C. Most cases of mild diarrheal disease do not require laboratory studies to determine the etiology. In moderate to severe diarrhea with fever or pus, a stool culture for bacterial pathogens (Salmonella, Shigella, Campylobacter) is submitted. If antibiotics were used recently, stool should be sent for Clostridium difficile toxin.

V. **Laboratory evaluation of acute diarrhea**
   A. **Fecal leukocytes** is a screening test which should be obtained if moderate to severe diarrhea is present. Numerous leukocytes indicate Shigella, Salmonella, or Campylobacter jejuni.
   B. **Stool cultures for bacterial pathogens** should be obtained if high fevers, severe or persistent (>14 d) diarrhea, bloody stools, or leukocytes are present.
   C. **Examination for ova and parasites** is indicated for persistent diarrhea (>14 d), travel to a high-risk region, gay males, infants in day care, or dysentery.
   D. **Blood cultures** should be obtained prior to starting antibiotics if severe diarrhea and high fever is present.
   E. **E coli 0157:H7 Cultures.** Enterotoxigenic E coli should be suspected if there are bloody stools with minimal fever, or when diarrhea follows hamburger consumption, or when hemolytic uremic syndrome is diagnosed.
   F. **Clostridium difficile cytotoxin** should be obtained if diarrhea follows use of an antimicrobial agent.
   G. **Rotavirus antigen test (Rotazyme)** is indicated for hospitalized children <2 years old with gastroenteritis. The finding of rotavirus eliminates the need for antibiotics.

VI. **Treatment of acute diarrhea**
   A. **Fluid and electrolyte resuscitation**
      1. **Oral rehydration.** For cases of mild to moderate diarrhea in children, Pedialyte or Ricelyte should be administered. For adults with diarrhea, flavored soft drinks with saltine crackers are usually adequate.
      2. **Intravenous hydration** should be used if oral rehydration is not possible.
   B. **Diet**. Fatty foods should be avoided. Well-tolerated foods include complex carbohydrates (rice, wheat, potatoes, bread, and cereals), lean meats, yogurt, fruits, and vegetables. Diarrhea often is associated with a reduction in intestinal lactase. A lactose-free milk preparation may be substituted if lactose intolerance becomes apparent.

VII. **Antimicrobial treatment of acute diarrhea**
   A. **Empiric drug therapy**
      1. **Febrile dysenteric syndrome**
         a. If diarrhea is associated with high fever and stools containing mucus

and blood, empiric antibacterial therapy should be given for Shigella or Campylobacter jejuni.

   b. Norfloxacin (Noroxin) 400 mg bid, ciprofloxacin (Cipro) 500 mg bid, ofloxacin (Floxin) 300 mg bid for 3-5 days.
2. **Travelers' diarrhea.** Adults are treated with norfloxacin 400 mg bid, ciprofloxacin 500 mg bid, or ofloxacin 300 mg bid for 3 days.

References: See page 195.

Chronic Diarrhea

Diarrhea is considered chronic if it occurs acutely, subsides, and then returns, or if it lasts longer than 2 weeks.

I. Clinical evaluation of chronic diarrhea
   A. Initial evaluation should determine the characteristics of the diarrhea, including volume, mucus, blood, flatus, cramps, tenesmus, duration, frequency, effect of fasting, stress, and the effect of specific foods (eg, dairy products, wheat, laxatives, fruits).
   B. Secretory diarrhea
      1. Secretory diarrhea is characterized by large stool volumes (>1 L/day), no decrease with fasting, and a fecal osmotic gap <40.
      2. **Evaluation of secretory diarrhea** consists of a giardia antigen, Entamoeba histolytica antibody, Yersinia culture, fasting serum glucose, thyroid function tests, and a cholestyramine (Cholybar, Questran) trial.
   C. Osmotic diarrhea
      1. Osmotic diarrhea is characterized by small stool volumes, a decrease with fasting, and a fecal osmotic gap >40. Postprandial diarrhea with bloating or flatus also suggests osmotic diarrhea. Ingestion of an osmotically active laxative may be inadvertent (sugarless gum containing sorbitol) or covert (with eating disorders).
      2. **Evaluation of osmotic diarrhea**
         a. Trial of lactose withdrawal.
         b. Trial of an antibiotic (metronidazole) for small-bowel bacterial overgrowth.
         c. Screening for celiac disease (anti-endomysial antibody, antigliadin antibody).
         d. Fecal fat measurement (72 hr) for pancreatic insufficiency.
         e. Trial of fructose avoidance.
         f. Stool test for phenolphthalein and magnesium if laxative abuse is suspected.
         g. Hydrogen breath analysis to identify disaccharidase deficiency or bacterial overgrowth.
   D. Exudative diarrhea
      1. Exudative diarrhea is characterized by bloody stools, tenesmus, urgency, cramping pain, and nocturnal occurrence. It is most often caused by inflammatory bowel disease, which may be indicated by the presence of anemia, hypoalbuminemia, and an increased sedimentation rate.
      2. **Evaluation of exudative diarrhea** consists of a complete blood cell count, serum albumin, total protein, erythrocyte sedimentation rate, electrolyte measurement, Entamoeba histolytica antibody titers, stool culture, Clostridium difficile antigen test, ova and parasite testing, and flexible sigmoidoscopy and biopsies.

References: See page 195.

Anorectal Disorders

I. Hemorrhoids
  A. Hemorrhoids are dilated veins located beneath the lining of the anal canal. Internal hemorrhoids are located in the upper anal canal. External hemorrhoids are located in the lower anal canal.
  B. Internal hemorrhoids become symptomatic when constipation causes disruption of the supporting tissues and resultant prolapse of the dilated anal veins. The most common symptom of internal hemorrhoids is painless rectal bleeding, which is usually bright red and ranges from a few drops to a spattering stream at the end of defecation. If internal hemorrhoids remain prolapsed, a dull aching may occur. Blood and mucus stains may appear on underwear, and itching in the perianal region is common.

Classification of Internal Hemorrhoids		
Grade	Description	Symptoms
1	Non-prolapsing	Minimal bleeding
2	Prolapse with straining, reduce when spontaneously prolapsed	Bleeding, discomfort, pruritus
3	Prolapse with straining, manual reduction required when prolapsed	Bleeding, discomfort, pruritus
4	Cannot be reduced when prolapsed	Bleeding, discomfort, pruritus

  C. Management of internal hemorrhoids
    1. Grade 1 and uncomplicated grade 2 hemorrhoids are treated with avoidance of nonsteroidal anti-inflammatory drugs and dietary modification (increased fiber and fluids).
    2. Symptomatic grade 2 and grade 3 hemorrhoids. Treatment consists of hemorrhoid banding with an anoscope Major complications are rare and consist of excessive pain, bleeding, and infection.
    3. Grade 4 hemorrhoids require surgical hemorrhoidectomy.
  D. External Hemorrhoids
    1. External hemorrhoids occur most often in young and middle-aged adults, becoming symptomatic only when they become thrombosed.
    2. External hemorrhoids are characterized by rapid onset of constant burning or throbbing pain, accompanying a new rectal lump. Bluish skin-covered lumps are visible at the anal verge.
    3. Pain is maximal in the first 48 hours and decreases thereafter to minimal discomfort after the 4 days.
    4. Management of external hemorrhoids
      a. If patients are seen in the first 48 hours, the entire lesion can be excised in the office. Local anesthetic is infiltrated, and the thrombus and overlying skin are excised with scissors. The resulting wound heals by secondary intention.
      b. If thrombosis occurred more than 48 hours prior, spontaneous resolution should be permitted to occur.

II. Anal Fissures

A. An anal fissure is a longitudinal tear in the distal anal canal, usually in the posterior or anterior midline. Anal fissures may be associated with secondary changes such as a sentinel tag, hypertrophied anal papilla, induration of the edge of the fissure, and anal stenosis. A patient with multiple fissures, or whose fissure is not in the midline, is more likely to have Crohn's disease.

B. Anal fissures are caused by spasm of the internal anal sphincter. Risk factors include a low fiber diet and previous anal surgery.

C. Patients with anal fissures complain of perirectal pain which is sharp, searing or burning and is associated with defecation. Bleeding from anal fissures is bright red and not mixed with the stool.

D. **Treatment**

1. High fiber foods, warm sitz baths, stool softeners (if necessary), and daily application of 1% hydrocortisone cream to the fissure should be recommended. These simple measures may heal acute anal fissures within 3 weeks in 90% of patients.

2. **Lateral partial internal sphincterotomy** is indicated when 4 weeks of medical therapy fails. It consists of surgical division of a portion of the internal sphincter, and it is highly effective. Adverse effects include incontinence to flatus and stool.

III. Levator Ani Syndrome and Proctalgia Fugax

A. Levator ani syndrome refers to chronic or recurrent rectal pain, with episodes lasting 20 minutes or longer. Proctalgia fugax connotes anal or rectal pain, lasting for seconds to minutes and then disappearing for days to months.

B. Levator ani syndrome and proctalgia fugax are more common in patients under age 45, and psychological factors are not always present.

C. Levator Ani Syndrome is caused by chronic tension of the levator muscle. Proctalgia fugax is caused by rectal muscle spasm. Proctalgia fugax and levator ani syndrome have not been found to be of psychosomatic origin, although stressful events may trigger attacks.

D. **Diagnosis and clinical features**

1. Levator ani syndrome is characterized by a vague, indefinite rectal discomfort or pain. The pain is felt high in the rectum and is sometimes associated with a sensation of pressure.

2. Proctalgia fugax causes pain that is brief and self limited. Patients with proctalgia fugax complain of sudden onset of intense, sharp, stabbing or cramping pain in the anorectum.

3. In patients with levator ani syndrome, palpation of the levator muscle during digital rectal examination usually reproduces the pain.

E. **Treatment**

1. **Levator ani syndrome.** Treatment with hot baths, nonsteroidal anti-inflammatory drugs, muscle relaxants, or levator muscle massage is recommended. Levator muscle massage consisting of, deep, digital pressure over the puborectalis portion of the levator floor is effective in 50-60%. EMG-based biofeedback may provide improvement in pain.

2. **Proctalgia fugax.** For patients with frequent attacks, physical modalities such as hot packs or direct anal pressure with a finger or closed fist may alleviate the pain. Diltiazem or oral clonidine may provided relief.

IV. Pruritus Ani

A. Pruritus ani is characterized by the intense desire to scratch the skin around the anal orifice. It occurs in 1% of the population. Pruritus ani may be related to fecal leakage.

B. Patients report an escalating pattern of itching and scratching in the perianal region. These symptoms may be worse at night. Anal hygiene and dietary habits, fecal soiling, and associated medical conditions should be sought.

C. Examination reveals perianal maceration, erythema, excoriation, and lichenification. The practitioner should perform a digital rectal examination and anoscopy to assess the sphincter tone and look for secondary causes of pruritus. Patients who fail to respond to 3 or 4 weeks of conservative treatment should undergo further investigations such as skin biopsy and sigmoidoscopy or colonoscopy.

D. Treatment and patient education

1. Patients should clean the perianal area with water following defecation, but avoid soaps and vigorous rubbing. Following this, the patient should dry the anus with a hair dryer or by patting gently with cotton. Between bowel movements a thin cotton pledget dusted with unscented cornstarch should be placed against the anus. A high fiber diet is recommended to regulate bowel movements and absorb excess liquid. All foods and beverages that may be exacerbating the itching should be eliminated.

2. Topical medications generally are not recommended because they may cause further irritation. If used, a bland cream such as zinc oxide or 1% hydrocortisone cream should be applied sparingly two to three times a day.

3. Systemic therapy with an antihistamine such as diphenhydramine (Benadryl) or hydroxyzine (Vistaril) may relieve the itching and allow the patient to sleep.

V. Perianal Abscess

A. The anal glands, located in the base of the anal crypts at the level of the dentate line, are the most common source of perianal infection. Acute infection presents as an abscess, and chronic infection results in a fistula.

B. The most common symptoms of perianal abscess are swelling and pain. Fevers and chills may occur. Perianal abscess is common in diabetic and immunosuppressed patients, and there is often a history of chronic constipation. A tender mass with fluctuant characteristics or induration is apparent on rectal exam

C. **Management of perianal abscess**. Perianal abscesses are treated with incision and drainage. If the abscess is small, incision and drainage using a local anesthetic is usually possible. Large abscesses require regional or general anesthesia. A cruciate incision is made close to the anal verge and the corners are excised to create an elliptical opening which promotes drainage. An antibiotic, such as Zosyn, Timentin, or Cefotetan, is administered.

D. About half of patients with anorectal abscesses will develop a fistula tract between the anal glands and the perianal mucosa, known as a fistula-in-ano. This complication manifests as either incomplete healing of the drainage site or recurrence. Healing of a fistula-in-ano requires a surgical fistulotomy.

References: See page 195.

Neurologic Disorders

Headache

Migraine affects 15% to 17% of women and 6% of men. Headaches can generally be grouped into three major categories: vascular, tension-type, and organic.

I. Clinical evaluation

    A. **Migraine** headaches are usually unilateral, and the acute attack typically lasts from 4 to 24 hours. Migraine headaches can occur with an aura or without an aura. Usually, the aura consists of focal neurologic symptoms starting 5 to 30 minutes before onset of an acute headache attack. Aura symptoms may continue for 15 to 30 minutes, resolving before the headache starts.

    B. The most common aura symptoms associated with migraine include scotomata (blind spots), teichopsia (fortification spectra, or the sensation of a luminous appearance before the eyes), photopsia (flashing lights), and paresthesias, as well as visual and auditory hallucinations, diplopia, ataxia, vertigo, syncope, and hyperosmia.

Features of Migraine Headache and Headache Caused by Serious Underlying Disease	
Migraine headache	**Headache caused by serious underlying disease**
History	
• Chronic headache pattern similar from attack to attack • Gastrointestinal symptoms • Aura, especially visual • Prodrome or postdrome	• Onset before puberty or after age 50 (tumor) • "Worst headache ever" (subarachnoid hemorrhage) • Headache occurring after exertion, sex, or bowel movement (subarachnoid hemorrhage) • Headache on rising in the morning (increased intracranial pressure, tumor) • Personality changes, seizures, alteration of consciousness (tumor) • Pain localized to temporal arteries or sudden loss of vision (giant cell arteritis) • Very localized headache (tumor, subarachnoid hemorrhage, giant cell arteritis)

Migraine headache	Headache caused by serious underlying disease
Physical examination	
• No signs of toxicity • Normal vital signs • Normal neurologic examination	• Signs of toxicity (infection, hemorrhage) • Fever (sinusitis, meningitis, or other infection) • Meningismus (meningitis) • Tenderness of temporal arteries (giant cell arteritis) • Focal neurologic deficits (tumor, meningitis, hemorrhage) • Papilledema (tumor)
Laboratory tests and neuroimaging	
• Normal results	• Erythrocyte sedimentation rate >50 mm/hr (giant cell arteritis) • Abnormalities on lumbar puncture (meningitis, hemorrhage) • Abnormalities on CT or MRI (tumor, hemorrhage, aneurysm)

C. Tension-type headache is a steady, aching pain of mild to moderate intensity, often characterized as a band-like pain around the head. Gastrointestinal and neurologic signs and symptoms usually do not occur.

D. Special attention should be paid to examining the fundus of the eye, assessing neck rigidity, and identifying any infectious process of the nose and throat. The temporal artery may appear dilated and pulsating. Neurologic symptoms should be evaluated with computed tomographic scanning. A lumbar puncture is appropriate if symptoms persist.

II. Treatment of migraine

A. **Dihydroergotamine**, which can be injected subcutaneously, intramuscularly or intravenously, or sprayed intranasally, is effective in treating migraine attacks. It is a weaker arterial vasoconstrictor than ergotamine and causes fewer adverse effects; it can cause diarrhea and muscle cramps. Dihydroergotamine nasal spray (Migranal) relieves migraine two hours in 50%.

B. **5-HT$_1$ Receptor Agonists ("Triptans")**

1. **Sumatriptan (Imitrex)** is available for subcutaneous self-injection, an oral formulation, and as a nasal spray. A selective serotonin-receptor agonist, it appears to be more effective than ergotamine. The injection and nasal spray begin to produce relief in 10 to 15 minutes, compared to one to two hours with the tablets. A subcutaneous injection produces relief in 70-80%. Sumatriptan nasal spray provides relief in about 60%. Oral sumatriptan is effective in 50-60%.

2. **Zolmitriptan (Zomig), naratriptan (Amerge), and rizatriptan (Maxalt).** Zolmitriptan and rizatriptan may have a more rapid onset of action than oral sumatriptan. Naratriptan, which has a longer half-life, has a slower onset of action. The rate of recurrence of migraine within 24 hours after treatment with a triptan is 30% to 40%; it may be slightly lower with naratriptan.

Drugs for Treatment of Migraine and Tension Headache

Drug	Dosage
NSAIDs	
Ibuprofen (Motrin)	400-800 mg, repeat as needed in 4 hr
Naproxen sodium (Anaprox DS)	550-825 mg, repeat as needed in 4 hr
5-HT₁ Receptor Agonists ("Triptans")	
Naratriptan (Amerge)	1- or 2.5-mg tablet, can be repeated 4 hours later (max 5 mg/24 hours)
Rizatriptan (Maxalt)	5- or 10-mg tablet or wafer (MLT); can be repeated in 2 hours (max 30 mg/24 hours)
Sumatriptan (Imitrex)	6 mg SC; can be repeated in 1 hour (max 2 injections/24 hours) 25, 50 or 100 mg PO; can be repeated in 2 hours (max 200 mg/24 hours) 5 or 20 mg intranasally; can be repeated after 2 hours (max 40 mg/24 hours)
Zolmitriptan (Zomig)	2.5 or 5 mg PO; can be repeated in 2 hours (max 10 mg/24 hours)
Ergot Alkaloids	
Dihydroergotamine DHE 45 Migranal Nasal Spray	1 mg IM; can be repeated twice at 1-hour intervals (max 3 mg/attack) 1 spray (0.5 mg)/nostril, repeated 15 minutes later (2 mg/dose; max 3 mg/24 hours)
Ergotamine 1 mg/caffeine 100 mg (Ercaf, Gotamine , Wigraine)	2 tablets PO, then 1 q30min, x 4 PRN (max 6 tabs/attack)
Ergotamine (Ergomar)	2-mg sublingual tablet, can be repeated q30min x 2 PRN (max 3 tabs/attack)
Ergotamine 2 mg/caffeine 100 mg (Cafergot)	One rectal suppository; can be repeated once, 1 hour later
Butalbital combinations	
Aspirin 325 mg, caffeine 40 mg, butalbital 50 mg (Fiorinal)	2 tablets, followed by 1 tablet q4-6h as needed
Acetaminophen 325 mg, caffeine 40 mg, butalbital 50 mg (Esgic, Fioricet)	2 tablets, followed by 1 tablet q4-6h as needed
Acetaminophen 325 mg, butalbital 50 mg (Phrenilin)	2 tablets, followed by 1 tablet as q4-6h needed

Drug	Dosage
Isometheptene combination	
Isometheptene 65 mg, acetaminophen 325 mg, dichloralphenazone 100 mg (Midrin)	2 tablets, followed by 1 tablet as needed q4-6h prn
Opioid Analgesics	
Butorphanol (Stadol NS)	One spray in one nostril; can be repeated in the other nostril in 60-90 minutes; the same two-dose sequence can be repeated in 3 to 5 hours

Drugs for Prevention of Migraine	
Drug	**Dosage**
Propranolol (Inderal)	80 to 240 mg/day, divided bid, tid or qid
Timolol (Blocadren)	10 to 15 mg bid
Divalproex sodium (Depakote)	250 mg bid or tid
Amitriptyline (Elavil)	10-150 mg qhs

C. **Prophylaxis against migraine**
   1. Patients with frequent or severe migraine headaches or those refractory to symptomatic treatment may benefit from prophylaxis. Menstrual or other predictable migraine attacks may sometimes be prevented by a brief course of ergotamine or an NSAID, such as naproxen sodium, taken for several days before and during the first few days of menstruation.
   2. **Beta-adrenergic blocking agents** are used most commonly for continuous prophylaxis. Propranolol, timolol, metoprolol (Lopressor), nadolol (Corgard, and others) and atenolol (Tenormin) have been effective.
   3. **Valproate (Depakote)**, an anticonvulsant, has been effective in decreasing migraine frequency. Its effectiveness was equal to that of propranolol. Adverse effects include nausea, weight gain and fatigue. Valproate taken during pregnancy can cause congenital abnormalities.
   4. **Tricyclic antidepressants** can prevent migraine and may be given concurrently with other prophylactic agents, but they often cause weight gain. Amitriptyline (Elavil) in a dosage ranging from 10 to 150 mg/day is commonly used.

References: See page 195.

Vertigo

The clinical evaluation of vertigo begins with the patient's description of symptoms and the circumstances in which they occur. Many drugs can cause dizziness. Common nonvestibular causes (eg, hyperventilation, orthostatic hypotension, panic disorder) are often diagnosed.

Types of dizziness according to clinical features

Type	Common description	Mechanism	Common causes	Focus of diagnostic workup
Vertigo	Spinning, whirling, tilting, veering, drunkenness	Imbalance in tonic vestibular signals	Benign positional vertigo, vestibular neuritis, Meniere's disease, migraine, vertebrobasilar insufficiency	Vestibular system
Near faint	Light-headedness, swimming sensation, blackout spells	Decreased oxygen supply to brain	Hyperventilation, orthostatic hypotension, vasovagal episodes, cardiac arrhythmia	Cardiovascular system
Hypoglycemia-induced	Light-headedness, disorientation, confusion	Decreased blood glucose level Increased catecholamines	Use of insulin, alcoholism, insulin-secreting tumor	Appropriate metabolic system
Psycho-physiology-induced	Disorientation, being "spaced out"	Impaired central integration	Anxiety, phobia, panic disorder	Psychiatric disorder
Disequilibrium	Unsteadiness, heavy-headedness	Sensorimotor impairment	Ototoxicity, peripheral neuropathy, multi-infarcts, cerebellar degeneration	Sensorimotor systems

Drugs Associated with Dizziness

Class of drug	Type of dizziness	Mechanism
Alcohol	Positional vertigo	Specific-gravity difference in endolymph vs cupula
Intoxication	CNS depression	Disequilibrium Cerebellar dysfunction
Tranquilizers	Intoxication	CNS depression
Anticonvulsants	Intoxication Disequilibrium	CNS depression Cerebellar dysfunction
Antihypertensives	Near faint	Postural hypotension

Class of drug	Type of dizziness	Mechanism
Aminoglycosides	Vertigo Disequilibrium Oscillopsia	Asymmetric hair-cell loss Vestibulospinal reflex loss Vestibulo-ocular reflex loss

III. Benign positional vertigo
   A. Benign positional vertigo is the most common cause of vertigo. Patients have brief episodes with positional change, typically when turning over in bed, getting out of bed, or bending over and straightening up. It is most common in older people.
   B. Diagnosis is by the Dix-Hallpike maneuver: fatigable, torsional, vertical, paroxysmal positional nystagmus resulting from a rapid change from the sitting to the head-hanging position. Benign positional vertigo is caused by calcium within the posterior semicircular canal.
IV. Acute unilateral vestibulopathy is characterized by acute onset of vertigo, nausea, and vomiting lasting for several days, not associated with auditory or neurologic symptoms. Most patients gradually improve over a few weeks, but older patients can have persistent symptoms for months. About half of patients report having had a recent viral upper respiratory tract infection.
V. Chronic bilateral vestibulopathy
   A. Chronic bilateral vestibulopathy presents with nonspecific dizziness and disequilibrium. Oscillopsia (an illusion that the environment is moving when the head is moved) is common.
   B. The most common cause is ototoxicity from aminoglycoside use. Aminoglycosides can produce both auditory and vestibular damage.
VI. Meniere's disease
   A. Meniere's disease is characterized by vertigo, hearing loss, and tinnitus. Most patients also experience a sense of fullness and pressure in the ear. Tinnitus is described as a roaring sound.
   B. Episodes occur at irregular intervals for years, often with periods of remission. Eventually, severe permanent hearing loss develops. The cause is an increase in the volume of endolymph.
VII. Migraine
   A. Vertigo is a common symptom of migraine, occurring in about 25% of migraineurs, either along with headache or in isolated episodes.
   B. Migraine-associated vertigo is usually associated with an aura and is followed by a unilateral throbbing headache. Long-standing motion sickness and a family history of migraine point to migraine.
VIII. Vertebrobasilar insufficiency
   A. Cerebrovascular disease is a common cause of vertigo in older patients, resulting from ischemia of the labyrinth and brain stem caused by vertebrobasilar circulation insufficiency. Vertigo has an abrupt onset, lasts for several minutes, and is accompanied by nausea, vomiting, and severe imbalance. Associated symptoms include visual blurring or blackouts, diplopia, drop attacks, weakness and numbness of the extremities, and headache.
   B. Atherosclerosis of the subclavian, vertebral, and basilar arteries is the most common cause. Risk factors include coronary artery disease, hypertension, diabetes mellitus, and hyperlipidemia. In young patients without obvious risk factors for atherosclerosis, traumatic dissection and systemic illness (eg, arteritis, hypercoagulation syndromes) should be considered.
   C. Magnetic resonance imaging is the study of choice to identify occlusive disease in the vessels of the neck and base of the brain.
IX. Treatment of vertigo
   A. A vestibular exercise program should be instituted as soon as possible.

While nystagmus is present, patients should attempt to focus the eyes and should move and hold them in the direction that provokes the most dizziness. When nystagmus has diminished to the point that the patient can clearly focus on a target in all directions, eye-head coordination exercises should be started. A useful exercise is to stare at a target while oscillating the head from side to side and up and down.

Treatment of Vertigo

Cause	Treatment
Benign positional vertigo	Maneuver to remove debris from semicircular canal
Acute unilateral	Antivertiginous drugs for first few days; vestibular rehabilitation
Chronic bilateral	Discontinuation of ototoxic agent; vestibular rehabilitation
Meniere's disease	Low-salt diet (1-2 g sodium daily) with diuretic; antivertiginous drugs; surgery in intractable cases
Migraine	Control of potential triggers (eg, foods, stress); antimigraine drugs (beta blockers)
Vertebrobasilar insufficiency	Antiplatelet drug (aspirin or ticlopidine); anticoagulant (heparin or warfarin [Coumadin]) if spells continue

Antivertiginous and Antiemetic Drugs

Classes and agents	Dosage	Comments
Antihistamines		
Dimenhydrinate (Benadryl)	50 mg PO q4-6h or 100-mg supp. q8h	Available without prescription, mild sedation, minimal side effects
Meclizine (Antivert)	25-50 mg PO q4-6h	Mild sedation, minimal side effects
Promethazine (Phenergan)	25-50 mg PO, IM, or suppository q4-6h	Good for nausea, vertigo, more sedation, extrapyramidal effects
Monoaminergic agents		
Amphetamine	5 or 10 mg PO q4-6h	Stimulant, can counteract sedation of antihistamines, anxiety
Ephedrine	25 mg PO q4-6h	Available without prescription
Benzodiazepine		
Diazepam (Valium)	5 or 10 mg PO q6-8h	Sedation, little effect on nausea
Phenothiazine		
Prochlorperazine (Compazine)	5-25 mg PO, IM, or suppository q4-6h	Good antiemetic; extrapyramidal side effects, particularly in young patients

Classes and agents	Dosage	Comments
Benzamide		
Metoclopramide (Reglan)	5-10 mg PO, IM, or IV q4-6h	Improves gastric emptying

References: See page 195.

Seizures and Epilepsy

Epilepsy is defined as the tendency to have recurrent, unprovoked seizures. The disorder has a prevalence of about 0.5 percent. Males are affected more often than females.

I. **Seizure classification**
   A. Seizures are divided into three classes: generalized, partial, and unclassified. Generalized seizures are further divided into absence seizures, myoclonic seizures, clonic seizures, tonic seizures, tonic-clonic seizures, and atonic seizures.
   B. Partial seizures are divided into simple partial seizures (consciousness is not impaired), complex partial seizures (consciousness is impaired), and partial seizures evolving to secondarily generalized seizures.

II. **Etiology**
   A. The cause of seizures may be described as either idiopathic, acute symptomatic, or remote symptomatic. Acute symptomatic seizures occur within three months of an active process such as a central nervous system infection, vascular disease, neoplasm, metabolic encephalopathy, toxin, drugs, eclampsia or trauma. Remote symptomatic seizures occur as a result of acquired brain injuries, such as congenital CNS disorders, asphyxia, hypoxia or ischemic events, cerebrovascular disease, resolved CNS infection, stroke, trauma, inborn errors of metabolism, or Alzheimer's or Pick's disease.
   B. The majority of seizures are classified as partial or secondarily generalized, and the etiology of the majority of seizures is idiopathic.
   C. Human immunodeficiency virus (HIV) infection may cause new-onset seizures. In patients with a seizure and risk factors for HIV infection, 8.2% may be infected with HIV.

III. **Clinical evaluation**
   A. The patient will be unable to recall the event. An attempt should be made to obtain information from an observer. A description of the motor activity, premonitory symptoms, postictal state, tongue-biting, incontinence and provoking factors should be sought.
   B. A history of systemic illness, drug use or abuse, pregnancy, mental retardation, developmental history, head trauma, altered mental function, focal weakness, risk factors for HIV infection, and a family history of seizure disorder should be evaluated.
   C. **Differentiation of seizures from similar clinical entities**
      1. Seizures are usually abrupt in onset.
      2. Seizures generally last from 90 to 120 seconds.
      3. Seizures are accompanied by an altered level of consciousness (except in partial simple seizures).
      4. Seizures exhibit purposeless, involuntary activity.
      5. Seizures are accompanied by a postictal state and amnesia regarding the event.
      6. Seizures are paroxysmal and stereotypic.
      7. The most common entity that is confused with epileptic seizures is

syncope. Repetitive clonic, myoclonic or dystonic movements commonly occur after fainting. These movements, however, rarely persist beyond five to 10 seconds and do not exhibit the progression from tonic to clonic phase seen in seizures.

Age-Related Causes of Seizures in Decreasing Order of Frequency

Adults 21 to 65 years of age	Adults 65 years of age and older
Alcohol withdrawal	Cerebrovascular
Toxins or drugs	Trauma
Tumor	Tumor
Trauma	Infection
Psychogenic	Alcohol withdrawal
Genetic	Toxins or drugs
Infection	Drug withdrawal
Cerebrovascular	Hypoxia
Metabolic	Metabolic
Hypoxia	Hypertensive encephalopathy
Renal failure	Hyperosmolar state
Hyperosmolar state (hyperglycemia)	Renal failure
Collagen vascular disease	Hepatic failure
Eclampsia	Degenerative
Multiple sclerosis	Factitious
Degenerative	Idiopathic
Hypertensive encephalopathy	
Idiopathic	

Conditions That May Be Confused with Seizures

Syncope	Migraine
Hypotension	Sleep disorders (eg, cataplexy, narcolepsy)
Metabolic conditions (eg, hypoglycemia)	Fluctuating delirium
Cardiac disease (arrhythmias, hypoperfusion)	Paroxysmal vertigo
	Episodic movement disorders
Cerebrovascular disease (transient ischemic attacks)	Psychogenic seizures
	Panic disorder

D. **Physical and neurologic examination** should assess signs of systemic illness, dysmorphic features, needle tracks and sclerosed veins (drug abuse), focal neurologic deficits, orthostatic blood pressure changes, cardiac murmurs, arrhythmias, and bruits.

IV. **Diagnostic Evaluation**
   A. **Laboratory evaluation** includes a complete blood count, electrolytes, calcium, magnesium, phosphorus, blood urea nitrogen, creatinine and glucose. Toxicology screen and evaluation of hepatic function should be considered.
   B. **Lumbar puncture** is essential when meningitis or encephalitis is suspected, as well as in immunocompromised patients.
   C. **Brain imaging.** All patients who experience a seizure should undergo brain imaging to detect underlying tumor, abscess, vascular malformation, stroke, or traumatic injury. In nonurgent cases, the imaging modality of choice is magnetic resonance imaging (MRI), since it is more sensitive than computed tomography (CT). In patients presenting with a seizure and new focal deficits, persistent altered mental status, fever, recent trauma, persistent headache, cancer, treatment with anticoagulation or an

immunocompromised state, emergent neuroimaging is recommended with a CT scan because CT has superior ability in the detection of acute hemorrhage.

D. **Electroencephalography (EEG).** Generalized spike-and-wave discharges are associated with generalized epilepsy. Focal discharges are associated with partial seizures. The presence of epileptiform abnormalities on EEG has a recurrence risk of 83%, compared with 41% with nonspecific abnormalities and 12 percent with a normal EEG.

V. **Treatment of Epilepsy**

A. Ongoing antiepileptic therapy is not usually indicated for patients with a single seizure. The decision to initiate antiepileptic therapy is based on the likelihood of recurrent seizures.

Epilepsy Syndromes	
Generalized	**Partial Seizures**

Seizure types: Absence, myoclonic, tonic-clonic
Neurologic examination: Normal
Neuroimaging: Normal
EEG: Normal background with fast (3 to 6 Hz) generalized spike-and-wave discharges
Examples:
    Childhood absence epilepsy
    Juvenile myoclonic epilepsy
    Epilepsy with generalized tonic-clonic seizures
Treatment: Valproate (Depakote), ethosuximide (Zarontin) (effective for absence seizures only), lamotrigine (Lamictal), topiramate (Topamax), felbamate (Felbatol)
	Seizure types: Simple partial (awareness unimpaired), complex partial (awareness impaired), secondarily generalized tonic-clonic
	Neurologic examination: Focal abnormalities common
	EEG: Normal or abnormal background with focal or multifocal epileptiform discharges
	Examples:
	    Temporal lobe epilepsy
	    Frontal lobe epilepsy
	Treatment: Carbamazepine (Tegretol), phenytoin (Dilantin), valproate (Depakote), new agents gabapentin, lamotrigine, tiagabine, topiramate, felbamate, vagus nerve stimulator, resective surgery

B. **Serum drug levels** are useful for documenting the level corresponding to the maximum tolerated dosage of antiepileptic medication and assessing medication status and patient compliance when a breakthrough seizure has occurred.

C. **Complete blood cell count with differential and platelet count, electrolytes and liver enzymes** should be obtained before instituting antiepileptic medication.

Seizure Drugs

Drug	Typical adult starting dosage	Typical increment and rate of increase	Most common dose-related adverse effects	Nondose-related and idiosyncratic reactions
Carbamazepine (Tegretol) (Tegretol-XR) (Carbatrol)	200 mg bid [100, 200] 200 mg bid [100, 200, 400] 200 mg bid [200, 300]	200 mg/week (taken tid-qid) 200 mg/week (taken bid) 200 mg/week (taken bid)	Dizziness, somnolence, ataxia, nausea, vomiting, diplopia, blurred vision	Hyponatremia, rash, Stevens-Johnson syndrome, leukopenia, aplastic anemia, agranulocytosis, transaminitis, hepatic failure
Ethosuximide (Zarontin)	250 mg qd-bid [250]	250 mg/week	Anorexia, nausea, vomiting, drowsiness, headache, dizziness	Rash, Stevens-Johnson syndrome, hemopoietic complications
Felbamate (Felbatol)	400 mg tid [400, 600]	400 to 600 mg/week	Anorexia, vomiting, insomnia, nausea, headache, dizziness	Aplastic anemia, hepatic failure
Gabapentin (Neurontin)	300 mg qd-tid [100, 300, 400]	300 mg/week (taken tid-qid)	Somnolence, dizziness, ataxia, fatigue	Rash, weight gain, behavior changes, peripheral edema
Lamotrigine (Lamictal)	25 mg every other day [25, 100, 150, 200] (with valproate [Depakote]), to 25 mg bid (with carbamazepine, phenobarbital or phenytoin [Dilantin])	25 mg/2 weeks (taken bid)	Dizziness, ataxia, somnolence, headache, diplopia, blurred vision, nausea, vomiting, rash	Rash, Stevens-Johnson syndrome, transaminitis
Phenobarbital	100 mg qd [15, 30, 60, 100]	15 to 30 mg/week	Somnolence, cognitive and behavior effects	Rash, Stevens-Johnson syndrome, hemopoietic complications, transaminitis, hepatic failure

Drug	Typical adult starting dosage	Typical increment and rate of increase	Most common dose-related adverse effects	Nondose-related and idiosyncratic reactions
Phenytoin (Dilantin)	300 mg qd [30, 50, 100]	25 to 30 mg/week	Ataxia, diplopia, slurred speech, confusion	Rash, Stevens-Johnson syndrome, hemopoietic complications, gingival hyperplasia, coarsening of facial features, transaminitis, hepatic failure
Tiagabine (Gabatril)	4 mg qd [4, 12, 16, 20]	4 mg/week (taken two to four times a day)	Dizziness, nervousness, asthenia, confusion, tremor	Not established
Topiramate (Topamax)	25 mg bid [25, 100, 200]	50 mg/week	Somnolence, dizziness, ataxia, slurred speech, psychomotor slowing, cognitive problems	Anemia, acne, alopecia, weight loss, transaminitis, nephrolithiasis
Valproate (Depakote)	250 mg tid [125, 250, 500]	250 mg/week	Nausea, vomiting, tremor, thrombocytopenia	Weight gain, hair changes/loss, transaminitis, hepatic failure, rash, Stevens-Johnson syndrome

D. New Antiepileptic Agents
1. **Felbamate (Felbatol)** is useful as adjunctive treatment or monotherapy in partial seizures. It has been associated with fatal idiosyncratic reactions, aplastic anemia, and fulminant hepatic failure.
2. **Gabapentin (Neurontin)** is used as adjunctive therapy in partial seizures. It is well suited for patients in whom drug-drug interactions must be avoided.
3. **Lamotrigine (Lamictal)** is used as adjunctive treatment for partial seizures. It has a broad spectrum of antiepileptic activity. The agent is used as an alternative for partial or generalized seizures.
4. **Topiramate (Topamax)** is indicated for adjunctive therapy in partial seizures. It may also be effective in some generalized epilepsies. Cognitive effects and nephrolithiasis may occur.
5. **Tiagabine (Gabatril)** is useful as adjunctive therapy for partial seizures. Dizziness and nervousness may occur.
6. **Fosphenytoin (Cerebyx)**, a parenteral phenytoin prodrug, is easier to administer and better tolerated than phenytoin, and it can be administered IV or IM.
7. **Extended-release carbamazepine (Tegretol-XR)** allows twice-daily dosing and provides more consistent serum levels of carbamazepine.
8. **Valproate (Depacon)** is available in a parenteral preparation and is indicated as an intravenous alternative when oral valproate is not feasible.
9. **Diazepam rectal gel (Diastat)** is helpful in controlling acute repetitive seizures in patients with refractory epilepsy.

E. Vagus nerve stimulator
is a treatment for refractory partial seizures. A 50 percent reduction in seizure frequency occurs in 30 percent of patients.

F. Seizure surgery
should be considered for patients in whom antiepileptic drugs fail to completely control seizures. Up to 80 percent become seizure-free after surgery.

References: See page 195.

Alzheimer's Disease

Dementia is an acquired syndrome in which intellectual ability decreases to the point that it interferes with daily function. There are two major causes of dementia in older persons: Alzheimer's disease and vascular dementia. Approximately 60 percent of dementing illnesses are caused by Alzheimer's disease, 15 percent are caused by vascular dementia and many of the remainder involve concurrent Alzheimer's disease and vascular dementia ("mixed dementia").

I. Pathophysiology
A. **Alzheimer's disease** is associated with diffuse neuron injury and death, with senile plaques and neurofibrillary tangles. The average duration of the disease is 10 years, during which afflicted persons progress from mild memory loss to the need for 24-hour supervision to total dependency and death. Risk factors for Alzheimer's disease are age, a family history of the disease, and Down syndrome.

B. **Vascular dementia** is generally one of two types: multi-infarct dementia or subcortical vascular dementia. In multi-infarct dementia, the neurologic examination reveals focal, asymmetric abnormalities, and multiple strokes are evident on computed tomography (CT) or magnetic resonance imaging (MRI) of the brain. Subcortical vascular dementia (Binswanger's disease) is characterized by vascular disease that predominantly affects the midbrain.

II. Diagnostic evaluation

    A. Dementia should be suspected whenever an older person is reported to have gradually increasing difficulty in the ability to learn and retain new information, handle complex tasks, or reason. Difficulties with spatial ability and orientation, language and behavior are common. The degree of cognitive impairment should be evaluated with a Mini-Mental State Examination, and focal neurologic findings should be sought.

Diagnostic Criteria for Delirium, Dementia, Alzheimer's Disease and Vascular Dementia

Diagnostic criteria for delirium

A change in cognition or development of a perceptual disturbance is present and not explained by a preexisting, established or evolving dementia.

The disturbance developed over a short period of time (usually hours to days) and tends to fluctuate.

The level of consciousness (awareness of the environment) is disturbed or fluctuates.

There is evidence that a drug, acute illness or metabolic disturbance is present that could explain the change in cognition.

Diagnostic criteria for dementia

Cognitive impairment is present, as demonstrated by: (1) memory loss and (2) impairment of language, praxis, recognition or abstract thinking.

The cognitive impairment is chronic and progressive and has resulted in functional decline.

Delirium has been ruled out.

Diagnostic criteria for Alzheimer's disease

Dementia is present.

History, physical and mental status examinations are consistent with Alzheimer's disease.

Screening blood tests (CBC, BUN, calcium, liver function, thyroid function, vitamin B_{12}) and review of medications do not reveal any cause of cognitive impairment.

Brain imaging study (CT or MRI) is normal or shows atrophy.

Diagnostic criteria for vascular dementia

Dementia is present.

Two or more of the following are present: (1) focal neurologic signs on physical examination; (2) an onset that was abrupt, stepwise or stroke-related; (3) brain imaging study (CT or MRI) shows multiple strokes.

    B. Testing a blood sample for apolipoprotein E may be used as an adjunct to other diagnostic procedures; a positive test increases likelihood that the dementia is due to Alzheimer's disease.

    C. Physicians should rule out delirium and search for coexisting conditions that worsen dementia by reviewing medications, screening for depression, and ruling out nutritional deficiencies, diabetes mellitus, uremia, alterations in electrolytes and thyroid disease.

Medications That May Cause Cognitive Impairment	
Antiarrhythmic agents	Antineoplastic agents
Antibiotics	Antiparkinsonian agents
Anticholinergic agents	Corticosteroids
Anticonvulsants	Histamine H_2-receptor antagonists
Antidepressants	Immunosuppressive agents
Antiemetics	Muscle relaxants
Antihistamines/decongestants	Narcotic analgesics
Antihypertensive agents	Sedatives
Antimanic agents	

III. Use of medication to delay symptom progression

A. **Tacrine (Cognex) and donepezil (Aricept)** are available for the treatment of Alzheimer's disease. Metrifonate and rivastigmine are in development and testing. Effects are modest: a good response to either drug will return the patient's function to the level that was present between six and 12 months before medication was started. Beneficial effects on behavior symptoms have been reported, and the use of tacrine has been shown to delay nursing home placement.

B. **Estrogen replacement therapy** has a significant protective effect and may delay the expression of Alzheimer's disease.

C. **Nonsteroidal anti-inflammatory drugs (NSAIDs)** such as aspirin and ibuprofen have been associated with a lower incidence of dementia. Because of the risks of gastrointestinal and renal toxicity, these agents cannot be routinely recommended as a preventive measure against Alzheimer's disease.

D. **Vitamin E** supplementation may significantly slow the progression of moderate Alzheimer's disease. Vitamin E supplementation may be considered in persons with dementia or those who are at risk for the disease. Dosages of up to 2,000 IU daily are used.

E. **Ginkgo biloba extract** has been reported to delay symptom progression in dementia, but little is known about the long-term effects of the extract, and it can not be recommended.

Drug Treatments for Dementia			
Diagnosis	**Medication**	**Typical dosage**	**Comments**
Alzheimer's disease	Donepezil (Aricept)	5 to 10 mg once daily	Equal efficacy and fewer side effects than tacrine; elevated hepatic transaminase levels are rare; diarrhea and abdominal pain occur occasionally.
	Tacrine (Cognex)	10 mg four times daily, increase at 6-week intervals to 40 mg four times daily	Elevated hepatic transaminase levels are common; check ALT every 2 weeks during dosage titration.
	Ibuprofen (Motrin)	400 mg two to three times daily	Gastrointestinal or renal toxicity.

Diagnosis	Medication	Typical dosage	Comments
	Conjugated estrogens (Premarin)	0.625 mg daily	Prescribe for women; add cyclic progestin for patients with an intact uterus.
	Vitamin E	800 to 2,000 IU daily	Mild antioxidant effects.
Vascular dementia	Antihypertensive medication.	Maintain systolic blood pressure below 150 to 160 mm Hg	Treatment that lowers diastolic blood pressure below 85 to 90 may worsen cognitive impairment.
	Enteric-coated aspirin	81 to 325 mg daily	Consider warfarin (Coumadin) if atrial fibrillation is present.
	Vitamin E	800 to 2,000 IU daily	Mild anticoagulant effects.

IV. Management of behavior problems in Alzheimer's disease

A. Delusions are treated with an antipsychotic agent such as haloperidol (Haldol) or risperidone (Risperdal).

B. Agitation should be treated with a short-acting antianxiety agent such as lorazepam (Ativan) or buspirone (BuSpar).

C. Depression is managed with a selective serotonin reuptake inhibitor, beginning at one half the usual dosage. If sedation is also desirable, trazodone (Desyrel) is useful.

References: See page 195.

Endocrinologic, Hematologic and Rheumatologic Disorders

Diabetes

Up to 4 percent of Americans have diabetes. Vascular disease accounts for over 70 percent of deaths in adults with diabetes.

I. Classification and Pathophysiology
   A. **Type 1 diabetes mellitus** primarily occurs in children and adolescents. Patients with type 1 diabetes have an absolute deficiency of endogenous insulin and require exogenous insulin for survival.
   B. **Type 2 diabetes** accounts for 90% of individuals with diabetes mellitus, and the incidence increases in frequency with age, obesity and physical inactivity. The initial problem in type 2 diabetes is resistance to the action of insulin at the cellular level.
   C. Type 1 and type 2 diabetes are associated with serious micro- and macrovascular complications. Overall life expectancy is shortened by five to seven years, with vascular disease being the cause of death in over 70%.

Characteristics of Type 1 and Type 2 Diabetes		
Characteristic	Type 1	Type 2
Age at onset	Under age 30	Over age 30
Percentage of ideal body weight	Less than 120 percent	Greater than 120 percent
Treatment	Insulin required	Insulin may or may not be required
Percentage of all patients with diabetes	10 percent	90 percent
Family history of diabetes	Usually negative	Usually positive

II. Screening
   A. All adults should be screened for diabetes at regular intervals. Factors that confer an increased risk for development of diabetes include impaired glucose tolerance, hypertension, lipid disorders, coronary artery disease, obesity, and physical inactivity.
   B. A fasting plasma glucose test is recommended for screening. A level of 110 to 125 mg/dL is considered to represent "impaired fasting glucose, and a value of greater than or equal to 126 mg/dL, if confirmed on repeat testing, establishes the diagnosis of diabetes. If a patient is found to have a random plasma glucose level over 160 mg/dL, more formal testing with a fasting plasma glucose should be considered. In cases in which an initial abnormal value is not confirmed on repeat testing, a glucose tolerance test may be administered.

Criteria for Diagnosis of Diabetes in Nonpregnant Adults

Fasting plasma glucose 126 mg/dL or higher
or
Random plasma glucose 200 mg/dL or higher with symptoms of diabetes (fatigue, weight loss, polyuria, polyphagia, polydipsia)
or
Abnormal two-hour 75-g oral glucose tolerance test result, with glucose 200 mg/dL or higher at two hours
Any abnormal test result must be repeated on a subsequent occasion to establish the diagnosis

---

Classification of Metabolic Control in Patients with Diabetes

Test	Good	Acceptable	Action warranted
HbA1c (normal: less than 6 percent)	6 percent or less	7 percent or less	Greater than 8 percent
Blood pressure	Less than 130/80 mm Hg	Less than 130/85 mm Hg	Greater than 140/90 mm Hg
Triglycerides	Less than 150 mg/dL	Less than 200 mg/dL	Greater than 400 mg/dL
Low-density lipoprotein cholesterol	Less than 100 mg/dL	Less than 130 mg/dL	Greater than 130 mg/dL

III. Screening for microvascular complications

A. Retinopathy. Diabetic retinopathy and macular degeneration are the leading causes of blindness in diabetes. These complications affect nearly all patients with type 1 diabetes and 60% of those with type 2 disease of at least 20 years duration. Adults with diabetes should receive annual dilated retinal examinations beginning at the time of diagnosis. Patients with active retinal hemorrhage should not use aspirin or engage in heavy lifting or strenuous exercise.

B. Nephropathy

   1. Diabetes-related nephropathy affects 40% of patients with type 1 disease and 10-20% of those with type 2 disease of 20 or more years duration. Microalbuminuria of 30 to 300 mg/24 hours heralds the onset of nephropathy. Microalbuminuria can be detected with annual urine screening for albumin/creatinine ratio. Abnormal screening test results should be confirmed, and a 24-hour urine sample should be obtained for total microalbuminuria assay and evaluation for creatinine clearance.

   2. The clinical progression of nephropathy can be slowed by (1) administering ACE inhibitors, such as lisinopril, enalapril or captopril (Capoten), (2) controlling blood pressure to 130\185 mm Hg or lower, (3) promptly treating urinary tract infections, (4) smoking cessation, and (5) limiting protein intake to 0.6 g/kg/day.

C. Neuropathy

   1. **Peripheral neuropathy** affects many patients with diabetes and causes nocturnal or constant pain, tingling and numbness and confers an

increased risk for foot infections, foot ulcers, and amputation.

    2. The feet should be evaluated regularly for sensation, pulses and sores. Semmes-Weinstein 10-g monofilament testing may be performed to accurately assess sensation.

  D. Autonomic neuropathy is found in many patients with long-standing diabetes. This problem can result in diarrhea, constipation, gastroparesis, vomiting, orthostatic hypotension, and erectile or ejaculatory dysfunction. Initial management of diarrhea consists of sugar-free psyllium [e.g., Metamucil, Sugar Free), loperamide (e.g., Imodium), 2.0 mg twice/day, or diphenoxylate/atropine sulfate (e.g., Lomotil) 2.5 mg twice/day. Sildenafil (Viagra) is beneficial in patients with erectile dysfunction

IV. Pharmacotherapy of diabetes

  A. Insulin

    1. Insulin should be prescribed for all patients with type 1 diabetes and is beneficial in many individuals with type 2 diabetes. A general strategy is to provide long-acting insulin to meet basal requirements and supplement this regimen with rapid-acting insulin taken shortly before mealtimes.

    2. NPH insulin is a long-acting insulin, which may be injected once per day at bedtime or twice per day, with about two-thirds of the daily dose given before breakfast and one-third given before the evening meal. Insulin therapy may be initiated in patients using oral agents by continuing the oral medications and adding 10 units of NPH insulin at 10 p.m. or bedtime.

    3. Short-acting insulins include regular insulin and lispro insulin. Either of these agents may be used before meals to match insulin availability to glucose load. Lispro has a more rapid onset of action and is also more rapidly cleared; therefore, it can be injected immediately before eating.

Features of Insulin Therapy

Type of insulin	Onset of action	Peak action	Duration of action	Comments
Lispro	10 minutes	One hour	Two hours	Inject immediately before meal
Regular	30 minutes	Two to four hours	Six to eight hours	Inject 15 to 30 minutes before meals
NPH	Two to four hours	Six to eight hours	Eight to 14 hours	Inject twice daily or at bedtime

Commonly Used Insulin Regimens

1. **One shot per day:** NPH at bedtime.
2. **Two shots per day:** NPH plus regular before breakfast and NPH plus regular before the evening meal.
3. **Three shots per day:** NPH plus regular before breakfast, regular before lunch and NPH plus regular before the evening meal.

B. Oral hypoglycemic agents

1. Biguanides

  a. **Metformin (Glucophage)** is an extremely potent and useful agent for the treatment of type 2 diabetes. A decrease of 1.5 to 2 percent in HbA1c can often be achieved. Metformin acts by reducing insulin resistance. It rarely causes hypoglycemia.

  b. Initial dose is 500 mg qd taken with a meal and slowly increased; a common maintenance dose is 1,000 mg bid, with a maximum dose of 850 mg tid. Gradual dose escalation can help minimize gastrointestinal side effects; diarrhea usually resolves over time.

  c. Metformin can precipitate fatal lactic acidosis; therefore, the drug should not be used in patients with serum creatinine >1.5 mg/dL, liver problems, or alcoholism.

2. Sulfonylureas

  a. Sulfonylureas, such as glipizide (Glucotrol, Glucotrol XL), glyburide (DiaBeta, Micronase) and glimepiride (Amaryl), increase insulin secretion and may reduce insulin resistance. They are typically used twice per day (except for Glucotrol XL and Amaryl). They may precipitate hypoglycemia.

  b. If a patient's glycemic control objective cannot be met using a maximal dose of the sulfonylurea, a second oral agent (metformin) or insulin should be added. No rationale exists for substituting one sulfonylurea for another or for substituting metformin for a sulfonylurea as monotherapy.

Pharmacotherapy of Diabetes			
Agent	Starting dose	Maximum dose	Comments
Sulfonylureas Glipizide (Glucotrol) Glyburide (DiaBeta, Micronase) Glimepiride (Amaryl)	5 mg daily 2.5 mg daily 1 mg daily	20 mg twice daily 10 mg twice daily 8 mg daily	May cause hypoglycemia, weight gain. Maximum dose should be used only in combination with insulin therapy
Biguanide Metformin (Glucophage)	500 mg daily	850 mg three times daily	Do not use if serum creatinine is greater than 1.4 mg/dL in women or 1.5 mg/dL in men or in the presence of heart failure, chronic obstructive pulmonary disease or liver disease; may cause lactic acidosis
Thiazolidine-dione Troglitazone (Rezulin)	200 mg daily	600 mg daily	Check bilirubin and liver function test results every two weeks for first six months; may cause hypoglycemia, weight gain
Alpha-glucosi-dase inhibitor Acarbose (Precose)	25 mg daily	100 mg three times daily	Flatulence; start at low dose to minimize side effects; take at mealtimes

Agent	Starting dose	Maximum dose	Comments
Meglitamide Repaglinide (Prandin)	0.5 mg before meals	4 mg three to four times daily	Mechanism of action similar to that of sulfonylureas; may cause hypoglycemia; take at mealtimes

3. **Troglitazone (Rezulin)**
   a. This agent is associated with weight gain and hypoglycemia. Starting dose is 200 mg once per day, which may be slowly increased to up to 600 mg once per day. Troglitazone should be administered with a meal and is often taken with breakfast. Metformin is more potent and usually associated with less serious side effects; therefore, troglitazone is a second-line agent.
   b. Idiosyncratic hepatocellular injury and liver failure associated with mortality has been reported. Liver function testing (AST, alkaline phosphatase, LDH, bilirubin) is recommended every 2 weeks for 6 months after starting the medication and periodically thereafter.
4. **Repaglinide (Prandin)**
   a. This agent stimulates insulin secretion. Repaglinide is a rapid-acting agent. It is useful for reducing postprandial hyperglycemia.
   b. Repaglinide is available as 0.5-, 1.0- and 2.0-mg tablets. The starting dose is 0.5 mg, taken no more than 30 minutes before a meal. The major side effect is hypoglycemia.
5. **Alpha-glucosidase inhibitors**
   a. Alpha-glucosidase inhibitors, such as acarbose, impair digestion of carbohydrates, reducing the amount of sugar that is absorbed from the small intestine. These agents are less potent than metformin or sulfonylureas and are often associated with gastrointestinal side effects.
   b. **Acarbose (Precose)** may be useful in patients who fail to adhere to dietary recommendations and have resultant weight gain. Acarbose should be started at a dose of 25 mg with a single daily meal and gradually increased to 25 mg with every meal; the dosage should then be slowly increased to a maximum of 100 mg.
C. **Approach to therapy**
   1. **In patients who are obese and have normal renal function** and no contraindications, treatment with metformin may be started at 500 mg each day before breakfast for one week, followed by 500 mg taken before breakfast and before the evening meal. The dose should be adjusted as needed up to 1,000 mg each morning and 1,000 to 1,500 mg with the evening meal.
   2. **A sulfonylurea** (eg, glipizide [Glucotrol] at a starting dose of 2.5 mg with breakfast and increased as needed up to a maximum of 20 mg bid) may be added to metformin if necessary. Alternatively, a bedtime dose of NPH insulin (starting with 10 units and increasing by 2 or 3 units as needed) may be added.
   3. **If serum creatinine is greater than 1.5 mg/dL** or another contraindication exists, metformin should be avoided. In such cases, a sulfonylurea may initially be used, with bedtime NPH insulin, acarbose or troglitazone added.
D. **Self-monitoring of blood glucose**. When stable, self-monitoring of blood glucose is performed twice per day on alternate days, rotating among breakfast, lunch, dinner and bedtime checks. For patients receiving intensive therapy and those undergoing medication adjustments, more frequent monitoring is needed. Readings taken during the night or two hours after eating may uncover significant hyper- or hypoglycemia.

Routine Diabetes Care

History
Review physical activity, diet, self-monitored blood glucose readings, medications
Assess for symptoms of coronary heart disease
Evaluate smoking status, latest eye examination results, foot care

Physical examination
Weight
Blood pressure
Foot examination
Pulse
Sores or callus
Monofilament test for sensation
Insulin injection sites
Refer for dilated retinal examination annually

Laboratory studies
HbA1c every three to six months
Annual fasting lipid panel
Annual microalbuminuria screen
Annual serum creatinine

References: See page 195.

Anemia

The prevalence of anemia is about 29 to 30 cases per 1,000 females of all ages and six cases per 1,000 males under the age of 45, rising to a peak of 18.5 cases per 1,000 men over age 75. Deficiencies of iron, vitamin B12 and folic acid are the most common causes.

I. **Clinical manifestations.** Severe anemia may be tolerated well if it develops gradually. Patients with an Hb of less than 7 g/dL will have symptoms of tissue hypoxia (fatigue, headache, dyspnea, light-headedness, angina). Pallor, syncope and tachycardia may signal hypovolemia and impending shock.

II. **History and physical examination**
   A. The evaluation should determine if the anemia is of acute or chronic onset, and clues to any underlying systemic process should be sought. A history of drug exposure, blood loss, or a family history of anemia should be sought.
   B. Lymphadenopathy, hepatic or splenic enlargement, jaundice, bone tenderness, neurologic symptoms or blood in the feces should be sought.

III. **Laboratory evaluation**
   A. **Hemoglobin and hematocrit** serve as an estimate of the RBC mass. Immediately after acute blood loss, the Hb will be normal.
   B. **Reticulocyte count** reflects the rate of marrow production of RBCs. Absolute reticulocyte count = (% reticulocytes/100) × RBC count. An increase of reticulocytes to greater than 100,000/mm³ suggests a hyperproliferative bone marrow.
   C. **Mean corpuscular volume (MCV)** often is used in classifying anemia (microcytic, normocytic, macrocytic).

Normal Hematologic Values			
Age of patient	Hemoglobin	Hematocrit (%)	Mean corpuscular volume (pm³)
One to three days	14.5-22.5 g per dL	45-67	95-121
Six months to two years	10.5-13.5 g per dL	33-39	70-86
12 to 18 years (male)	13.0-16.0 g per dL	37-49	78-98
12 to 18 years (female)	12.0-16.0 g per dL	36-46	78-102
>18 years (male)	13.5-17.5 g per dL	41-53	78-98
>18 years (female)	12.0-16.0 g per dL	36-46	78-98

IV. Iron deficiency anemia

A. Iron deficiency is the most common cause of anemia. In children, the deficiency is typically caused by diet. In adults, the cause should be considered to be a result of chronic blood loss until a definitive diagnosis is established.

B. **Laboratory results**
   1. The MCV is usually normal in early iron deficiency. As the hematocrit falls below 30%, hypochromic microcytic cells appear, followed by a decrease in the MCV.
   2. **A serum ferritin level** of less than 10 ng/mL in women or 20 ng/mL in men is indicative of low iron stores. A serum ferritin level of more than 200 ng/mL indicates adequate iron stores.

C. **Treatment of iron deficiency anemia**
   1. Ferrous salts of iron are absorbed much more readily and are generally preferred. Commonly available oral preparations include ferrous sulfate, ferrous gluconate and ferrous fumarate (Hemocyte). All three forms are well absorbed. Ferrous sulfate is the least expensive and most commonly used oral iron supplement.

Oral Iron Preparations			
Preparation	Elemental iron (%)	Typical dosage	Elemental iron per dose
Ferrous sulfate	20	325 mg three times daily	65 mg
Ferrous sulfate, exsiccated (Feosol)	30	200 mg three times daily	65 mg
Ferrous gluconate	12	325 mg three times daily	36 mg

Preparation	Elemental iron (%)	Typical dosage	Elemental iron per dose
Ferrous fumarate (Hemocyte)	33	325 mg twice daily	106 mg

2. For iron replacement therapy, a dosage equivalent to 150 to 200 mg of elemental iron per day is recommended.
3. Ferrous sulfate, 325 mg of three times a day, will provide the necessary elemental iron for replacement therapy. Hematocrit levels should show improvement within one to two months of initiation of therapy.
4. Depending on the cause and severity of the anemia, and on whether there is continuing blood loss, replacement of low iron stores usually requires four to six months of iron supplementation. A daily dosage of 325 mg of ferrous sulfate may be necessary for maintenance therapy.
5. **Side effects** from oral iron replacement therapy are common and include nausea, constipation, diarrhea and abdominal pain. To minimize side effects, iron supplements should be taken with food; however, this may decrease iron absorption by 40 to 66 percent. Changing to a different iron salt or to a controlled-release preparation may also reduce side effects.
6. For optimum delivery, oral iron supplements must dissolve rapidly in the stomach so that the iron can be absorbed in the duodenum and upper jejunum. Enteric-coated preparations are ineffective since they do not dissolve in the stomach.
7. Causes of resistance to iron therapy include continuing blood loss, ineffective intake and ineffective absorption. Continuing blood loss may be overt (eg, menstruation, hemorrhoids) or occult (e.g., gastrointestinal malignancies, intestinal parasites, nonsteroidal anti-inflammatory drugs).
   a. Ineffective iron intake may be the result of poor compliance because of gastrointestinal side effects. Iron uptake and absorption may be impaired by the use of antacids, H2-receptor blockers and proton pump inhibitors. Caffeinated beverages, particularly tea, will also reduce iron absorption.
   b. Ineffective absorption of iron may also be the result of malabsorption states, such as celiac disease, Crohn's disease or pernicious anemia.
   c. If the patient does not respond adequately to oral iron supplementation, parenteral treatment with iron dextran (Infed) should be considered.
   d. Unpredictable absorption and local complications of intramuscular administration make the intravenous route preferable for parenteral iron treatment. Parenteral iron dextran may be administered as a single dose. The total dosage required to replenish body stores is determined with the following formula: Dose of iron (mg) = 0.3 x body wt (lb) x (100 - {[Hb (g/dL)/14.8] x 100})
   e. **Injectable iron dextran**, containing 50 mg of iron per mL, is supplied in a 2-mL single-dose vial. Adverse reactions include headache, dyspnea, flushing, nausea and vomiting, fever, hypotension, seizures, urticaria, anaphylaxis and chest, abdominal or back pain. A small test dose (0.5 mL) should be given to determine whether an anaphylactic reaction will occur. If the patient tolerates the test dose, the full-dosage may then be given at a rate of 50 mg per minute, up to a total daily dosage of 100 mg.

V. Vitamin B12 deficiency anemia
   A. Since body stores of vitamin B12 are adequate for up to five years, deficiency is generally the result of failure to absorb it. Pernicious anemia, Crohn's disease and other intestinal disorders are the most frequent causes

of vitamin B12 deficiency.
  - **B.** Symptoms are attributable primarily to anemia, although glossitis, jaundice, and splenomegaly may be present. Vitamin B12 deficiency may cause decreased vibratory and positional sense, ataxia, paresthesias, confusion, and dementia. Neurologic complications may occur in the absence of anemia and may not resolve completely despite adequate treatment. Folic acid deficiency does not result in neurologic disease.
  - **C. Laboratory results**
    1. A macrocytic anemia usually is present, and leukopenia and thrombocytopenia may occur. Lactate dehydrogenase (LDH) and indirect bilirubin typically are elevated.
    2. Vitamin B12 levels are low. RBC folate levels should be measured to exclude folate deficiency.
  - **D. Treatment of vitamin B 12 deficiency anemia.** Intramuscular, oral or intranasal preparations are available for B 12 replacement. In patients with severe vitamin B12 deficiency, daily IM injections of 1,000 mcg of cyanocobalamin are recommended for five days, followed by weekly injections for four weeks. Hematologic improvement should begin within five to seven days, and the deficiency should resolve after three to four weeks.

Vitamin B12 and Folic Acid Preparations	
Preparation	**Dosage**
Cyanocobalamin tablets	1,000 µg daily
Cyanocobalamin injection	1,000 µg weekly
Cyanocobalamin nasal gel (Nascobol)	500 µg weekly
Folic acid (Folvite)	1 mg daily

VI. Folate deficiency anemia
  - **A.** Folate deficiency is characterized by megaloblastic anemia and low serum folate levels. Most patients with folate deficiency have inadequate intake. Lactate dehydrogenase (LDH) and indirect bilirubin typically are elevated, reflecting ineffective erythropoiesis and premature destruction of RBCs.
  - **B. RBC folate and serum vitamin B$_{12}$ levels** should be measured. RBC folate is a more accurate indicator of body folate stores than is serum folate, particularly if measured after folate therapy has been initiated.
  - **C. Treatment of folate deficiency anemia**
    1. A once-daily dosage of 1 mg of folic acid given PO will replenish body stores in about three weeks.
    2. Folate supplementation is also recommended for women of child-bearing age to reduce the incidence of fetal neural tube defects. Folic acid should be initiated at 0.4 mg daily before conception. Most prenatal vitamins contain this amount. Women who have previously given birth to a child with a neural tube defect should take 4 to 5 mg of folic acid daily.

References: See page 195.

Herniated Lumbar Disc

Symptoms of a herniated lumbar disc may often be difficult to distinguish from those of other spinal disorders or simple back strain

I. Clinical evaluation

  A. The most common levels for a herniated disc are L4-5 and L5-S1. The onset of symptoms is characterized by a sharp, burning, stabbing pain radiating down the posterior or lateral aspect of the leg, to below the knee. Pain is generally superficial and localized, and is often associated with numbness or tingling. In more advanced cases, motor deficit, diminished reflexes or weakness may occur.

  B. If a disc herniation is responsible for the back pain, the patient can usually recall the time of onset and contributing factors, whereas if the pain is of a gradual onset, other degenerative diseases are more probable than disc herniation.

  C. Rheumatoid arthritis often begins in the appendicular skeleton before progressing to the spine. Inflammatory arthritides, such as ankylosing spondylitis, cause generalized pain and stiffness that are worse in the morning and relieved somewhat throughout the day.

"Red Flags" for Potentially Serious Conditions	
Possible condition	Findings from the medical history
Fracture	• Major trauma (motor vehicle accident, fall from height) • Minor trauma or strenuous lifting in an older or osteoporotic patient
Tumor or infection	• Age >50 years or <20 years • History of cancer • Constitutional symptoms (fever, chills, unexplained weight loss) • Recent bacterial infection • Intravenous drug use • Immunosuppression (corticosteroid use, transplant recipient, HIV infection) • Pain worse at night or in the supine position
Cauda equina syndrome	• Saddle anesthesia • Recent onset of bladder dysfunction • Severe or progressive neurologic deficit in lower extremity

  D. Cauda equina syndrome. Only the relatively uncommon central disc herniation provokes low back pain and saddle pain in the S1 and S2 distributions. A central herniated disc may also compress nerve roots of the cauda equina, resulting in difficult urination, incontinence or impotence. If bowel or bladder dysfunction is present, immediate referral to a specialist is required for emergency surgery to prevent permanent loss of function.

  E. Low back strain should be differentiated from central herniated disc. Pain caused by low back strain is exacerbated during standing and twisting motions, whereas pain caused by central disc herniation is worse in positions (such as sitting) that produce increased pressure on the disc.

II. **Physical and neurologic examination of the lumbar spine**
   A. **External manifestations of pain**, including an abnormal stance, should be noted. The patient's posture and gait should be examined for sciatic list, which is indicative of disc herniation. The spinous processes and interspinous ligaments should be palpated for tenderness.
   B. **Range of motion** should be evaluated. Pain during lumbar flexion suggests discogenic pain, while pain on lumbar extension suggests facet disease. Ligamentous or muscular strain can cause pain when the patient bends contralaterally.
   C. **Motor, sensory and reflex function** should be assessed to determine the affected nerve root level. Muscle strength is graded from zero (no evidence of contractility) to 5 (complete range of motion against gravity, with full resistance).
   D. **Specific movements and positions that reproduce the symptoms** should be documented. The upper lumbar region (L1, L2 and L3) controls the iliopsoas muscles, which can be evaluated by testing resistance to hip flexion. While seated, the patient should attempt to raise each thigh while the physician's hands are placed on the leg to create resistance. Pain and weakness are indicative of upper lumbar nerve root involvement. The L2, L3 and L4 nerve roots control the quadriceps muscle, which can be evaluated by manually trying to flex the actively extended knee. The L4 nerve root also controls the tibialis anterior muscle, which can be tested by heel walking.
   E. **The L5 nerve root** controls the extensor hallucis longus, which can be tested with the patient seated and moving both great toes in a dorsiflexed position against resistance. The L5 nerve root also innervates the hip abductors, which are evaluated by the Trendelenburg test. This test requires the patient to stand on one leg; the physician stands behind the patient and puts his or her hands on the patient's hips. A positive test is characterized by any drop in the pelvis on the opposite side and suggests either L5 nerve root pathology.
   F. **Cauda equina syndrome** can be identified by unexpected laxity of the anal sphincter, perianal or perineal sensory loss, or major motor loss in the lower extremities.
   G. **Nerve root tension signs** are evaluated with the straight-leg raising test in the supine position. The physician raises the patient's legs to 90 degrees. Normally, this position results in only minor tightness in the hamstrings. If nerve root compression is present, this test causes severe pain in the back of the affected leg and can reveal a disorder of the L5 or S1 nerve root.
   H. **The most common sites for a herniated lumbar disc** are L4-5 and L5-S1, resulting in back pain and pain radiating down the posterior and lateral leg, to below the knee.
   I. **A crossed straight-leg raising test** may suggest nerve root compression. In this test, straight-leg raising of the contralateral limb reproduces more specific but less intense pain on the affected side. In addition, the femoral stretch test can be used to evaluate the reproducibility of pain. The patient lies in either the prone or the lateral decubitus position, and the thigh is extended at the hip, and the knee is flexed. Reproduction of pain suggests upper nerve root (L2, L3 and L4) disorders.
   J. **Nonorganic physical signs (Waddell signs)** may identify patients with pain of a psychologic or socioeconomic basis. These signs include superficial tenderness, positive results on simulation tests (ie, maneuvers that appear to the patient to be a test but actually are not), distraction tests that attempt to reproduce positive physical findings when the patient is distracted, regional disturbances that do not correspond to a neuroanatomic or dermatomal distribution and overreaction during the examination.

Location of Pain and Motor Deficits in Association with Nerve Root Involvement

Disc level	Location of pain	Motor deficit
T12-L1	Pain in inguinal region and medial thigh	None
L1-2	Pain in anterior and medial aspect of upper thigh	Slight weakness in quadriceps; slightly diminished suprapatellar reflex
L2-3	Pain in anterolateral thigh	Weakened quadriceps; diminished patellar or suprapatellar reflex
L3-4	Pain in posterolateral thigh and anterior tibial area	Weakened quadriceps; diminished patellar reflex
L4-5	Pain in dorsum of foot	Extensor weakness of big toe and foot
L5-S1	Pain in lateral aspect of foot	Diminished or absent Achilles reflex

III. Imaging of the herniated disc
A. The major finding on plain radiographs of patients with a herniated disc is decreased disc height. Radiographs have limited diagnostic value for herniated disc because degenerative changes are equally present in asymptomatic and symptomatic persons.

B. The gold standard for herniated disc is magnetic resonance imaging (MRI). MRI has the ability to demonstrate disc damage, including anular tears and edema. MRI can reveal bulging and degenerative discs in asymptomatic persons; therefore, any management decisions should be based on the clinical findings corroborated by diagnostic test results.

IV. Treatment of herniated disc
A. The majority of patients experience resolution of their symptoms regardless of the treatment method. About 70 percent of patients have a marked reduction in leg pain within four weeks of the onset of symptoms. Symptomatic treatment is recommended for patients with symptoms of herniated disc during the first six weeks of symptoms. Most patients with low back pain respond well to conservative therapy, including limited bed rest, exercise, NSAIDs and injections.

B. **Bed rest** in excess of two days is not associated with a better outcome and continuing to perform usual activities as tolerated leads to more rapid recovery than bed rest. Excessive bed rest can result in deconditioning, bone mineral loss and economic loss.

C. **Analgesics**
   1. Naproxen (Naprosyn) 500 mg followed by 250 mg PO tid-qid prn [250, 375,500 mg].
   2. Naproxen sodium (Aleve) 200 mg PO tid prn.
   3. Naproxen sodium (Anaprox) 550 mg, followed by 275 mg PO tid-qid prn.
   4. Ibuprofen (Motrin, Advil) 800 mg, then 400 mg PO q4-6h prn.

D. **Aerobic exercise** may strengthen the abdominal and back muscles, relieve symptoms, reduce weight and alleviate depression and anxiety.

E. **Trigger point injections** can provide extended relief for localized pain sources. An injection of 1 to 2 mL of 1 percent lidocaine (Xylocaine) without epinephrine is usually administered. Ultrasound (phonophoresis) or electricity (iontophoresis) over the injected area may provide additional relief. Epidural steroid injection therapy has been reported to be effective in patients with lumbar disc herniation with radiculopathy.

F. Indications for herniated disc surgery. While most patients with a herniated disc may be effectively treated conservatively. Indications for referral include the following: (1) cauda equina syndrome, (2) progressive neurologic deficit, (3) profound neurologic deficit and (4) severe and disabling pain refractory to four to six weeks of conservative treatment.

References: See page 195.

Osteoarthritis

Osteoarthritis affects about 2% to 6% of the general population. The loss of articular cartilage with associated remodeling of subchondral bone is the defining characteristic of osteoarthritis.

I. **Diagnosis**
   A. Osteoarthritis pain is described as deep, aching and poorly localized. Pain is typically of slow onset, initially occurring after activity, with relief after rest. In severe cases there is pain at rest.
   B. Joint stiffness is common in osteoarthritis, characteristically occurring upon awakening or after inactivity. The stiffness lasts for 20 to 30 minutes, in contrast to the prolonged joint stiffness with rheumatoid arthritis. In contrast to rheumatoid arthritis, inflammation is not a prominent finding in osteoarthritis. Signs of prominent inflammation, such as joint effusions and localized warmth, are suggestive of rheumatoid arthritis.
   C. Osteoarthritis most commonly affects the hands, spine, knees, and hips while involvement of the wrist, elbows and shoulders is uncommon.

II. **Diagnosis of osteoarthritis of the knee**
   A. Pain, usually with activity, is the characteristic early symptom of osteoarthritis of the knee. Joint stiffness, present after rest or inactivity, improves with activity. Joint range of motion should be assessed
   B. Rheumatoid arthritis can be distinguished from osteoarthritis by the pattern of symmetrical peripheral joint involvement and the presence of inflammation in rheumatoid arthritis.

III. **Diagnosis of osteoarthritis of the hip**
   A. Hip osteoarthritis presents as pain in the groin, although buttock or anterior thigh or ipsilateral knee pain may also be present. The pain is insidious in nature, typically progresses over a course of months to years, and is described as dull or aching.
   B. The patient's posture and gait should be carefully evaluated. The hip joint is palpated to detect signs of local inflammation. Tenderness over the greater trochanter suggests bursitis, while groin tenderness suggests adenopathy, infection or possible neoplasm. Patients with sciatic nerve involvement due to disc disease or osteoarthritis of the spine may describe tenderness over the course of the sciatic nerve. A positive straight leg raising test also suggests sciatica.
   C. X-ray findings include osteophyte formation and loss of articular cartilage (ie, joint space narrowing), progressing to total obliteration of the joint space in severe cases.

IV. **Nonpharmacologic management of osteoarthritis**
   A. Joint protection
      1. Activities designed to minimize pain and prevent further joint damage include the following:
         a. Avoiding prolonged periods in the same position.
         b. Good posture to reduce stress on joints.

        c. Maintaining range of motion (ROM).

        d. Good joint alignment; unloading painful joints.

    2. In patients with osteoarthritis of the hip or knee, use of a cane or crutch on the opposite side can reduce weight-bearing on the affected joint by 30% to 40%. In patients with osteoarthritis of the knee, bracing and shoe wedges may be helpful.

B. Exercise

    1. Range of motion, muscle strengthening, and endurance exercises focus on reducing pain and maintaining joint function. Aerobic exercises include walking, stationary bicycle riding and aquatic exercise.

    2. Strength and endurance training. Muscle disuse from inactivity quickly erodes strength. Isometric exercises that do not involve joint motion are the most commonly used in osteoarthritis.

    3. Thermal therapy, either hot or cold, is often used as an adjunct to exercise. Patients with acute pain may responds best to cold therapy, while chronic pain is best treated with superficial heat.

C. Obesity and weight-loss. A rational weight-loss program is a critical component for any obese patient with osteoarthritis of the knee or hip.

V. Pharmacological management of osteoarthritis

    A. Nonsteroidal anti-inflammatory drugs (NSAIDS)

        1. Drug selection

            a. There is little difference in the effectiveness of NSAIDs among patients; however, the effectiveness and side effects, particularly dyspepsia, may vary markedly from patient to patient.

Commonly Used NSAIDs

Product	Dosage Form	Dose
Ibuprofen (Motrin)	300, 400, 600, 800 mg tablets	400/600/800 mg tid-qid
Naproxen (Naprosyn)	250, 375, 500 mg tablets	250/375/500 mg bid
Naproxen (EC-Naprosyn)	375, 500 mg tablets	375/500 mg bid
Etodolac (Lodine)	200, 300 mg capsule, 400 mg tablet	200/300/400 mg bid-tid
Fenoprofen (Nalfon)	200, 300 mg pulvule 600 mg tablet	300-600 mg tid-qid
Ketoprofen (Orudis)	25, 50, 75 mg capsule	50 mg qid 75 mg tid
Flurbiprofen (Ansaid)	50, 100 mg tablet	50/100 mg bid-tid
Tolmetin (Tolectin)	200, 600 mg tablet 400 mg capsule	200/400/600 mg bid-tid in divided doses
Diclofenac sodium (Voltaren)	25, 50, 75 mg tablet	50 mg bid-tid 75 mg bid
Oxaprozin (DayPro)	600 mg tablet	600-1200 mg qd

Product	Dosage Form	Dose
Piroxicam (Feldene)	10, 20 mg tablet	20 mg qd
Ketoprofen extended release (Oruvail)	200 mg capsule	200 mg qd
Nabumetone (Relafen)	500, 750 mg tablet	1000-2000 mg qd

  2. **Gastrointestinal side effects**
     a. Gastrointestinal effects are the most common and clinically significant side effect of NSAIDs. GI effects range from dyspepsia to erosions to ulceration.
     b. Concomitant use of misoprostol may prevent NSAID-induced ulcers. Misoprostol should be considered for high-risk patients with a history of peptic ulcer disease or upper GI bleeding, or who are taking corticosteroids or anticoagulants.
     c. Omeprazole (Prilosec), has been shown to be effective in preventing ulcers in patients who are taking NSAIDs.
  3. **Renal toxicity**
     a. Renal effects are a major toxicity of NSAIDs. Therefore, elderly patients with preexisting renal impairment are at high risk for renal toxicities.
 B. **Cyclooxygenase-2 inhibitors**
  1. **Celecoxib (Celebrex)** is a nonsteroidal anti-inflammatory drug (NSAID) that inhibits prostaglandin synthesis by inhibition of cyclooxygenase-2 (COX-2); celecoxib decreases joint pain, tenderness, and swelling of arthritis and is comparable to NSAIDs. Unlike NSAIDS, celecoxib is not associated with peptic ulceration, and it does not affect platelet aggregation and bleeding time. Dosage is 200 mg per day administered as a single dose or as 100 mg twice per day. Celecoxib has been associated with five deaths due to hepatotoxicity.
  2. **Refocoxib (Vioxx)** is also a selective COX 2 inhibitor.
 C. **Other medical therapies for osteoarthritis of the knee**
  1. **Joint aspiration** followed by an intra-articular injection of steroids may provide pain relief.
  2. **Intra-articular hyaluronan** is an alternative to NSAID therapy in the treatment of osteoarthritis of the knee. Intra-articular hyaluronan for knee osteoarthritis reduces pain similarly to NSAIDs.
VI. **Surgical therapies.** Joint lavage and arthroscopic debridement are options for patients with osteoarthritis of the knee who have not responded to pharmacologic therapy. Carefully selected patients with osteoarthritis of the knee or hip may benefit from an osteotomy. Osteotomies can provide pain relief in patients who are not candidates for total joint arthroplasty.

References: See page 195.

Gout

Gout comprises a heterogeneous group of disorders characterized by deposition of uric acid crystals in the joints and tendons. Gout has a prevalence of 5.0 to 6.6 cases per 1,000 men and 1.0 to 3.0 cases per 1,000 women.
I. **Clinical features**
 A. **Asymptomatic hyperuricemia** is defined as an abnormally high serum

urate level, without gouty arthritis or nephrolithiasis. Hyperuricemia is defined as a serum urate concentration greater than 7 mg/dL. Hyperuricemia predisposes patients to both gout and nephrolithiasis, but therapy is generally not warranted in the asymptomatic patient.

B. Acute gout is characterized by the sudden onset of pain, erythema, limited range of motion and swelling of the involved joint. The peak incidence of acute gout occurs between 30 and 50 years of age. First attacks are monoarticular in 90 percent. In more than one half of patients, the first metatarsophalangeal joint is the initial joint involved, a condition known as podagra. Joint involvement includes the metatarsophalangeal joint, the instep/forefoot, the ankle, the knee, the wrist and the fingers.

C. Intercritical gout consists of the asymptomatic phase of the disease following recovery from acute gouty arthritis.

D. Recurrent gouty arthritis. Approximately 60 percent of patients have a second attack within the first year, and 78 percent have a second attack within two years.

E. Chronic tophaceous gout. Tophi are deposits of sodium urate that are large enough to be seen on radiographs and may occur at virtually any site. Common sites include the joints of the hands or feet. The helix of the ear, the olecranon bursa, and the Achilles tendon.

II. Diagnosis

A. Definitive diagnosis requires aspiration and examination of synovial fluid for monosodium urate crystals. Monosodium urate crystals are identified by polarized light microscopy.

B. If a polarizing microscope is not available, the characteristic needle shape of the monosodium urate crystals, especially when found within white blood cells, can be identified with conventional light microscopy. The appearance resembles a toothpick piercing an olive.

III. Treatment of gout

A. Asymptomatic hyperuricemia. Urate-lowering drugs should not be used to treat patients with asymptomatic hyperuricemia. If hyperuricemia is identified, associated factors such as obesity, hypercholesterolemia, alcohol consumption and hypertension should be addressed.

B. Acute gout

1. NSAIDs are the preferred therapy for the treatment of acute gout. Indomethacin (Indocin), ibuprofen (Motrin), naproxen (Naprosyn), sulindac (Clinoril), piroxicam (Feldene) and ketoprofen (Orudis) are effective. More than 90 percent of patients have a resolution of the attack occurs within five to eight days.

Drugs Used in the Management of Acute Gout		
Drug	**Dosage**	**Side effects/comments**
NSAIDS		
Indomethacin (Indocin)	25 to 50 mg four times daily	Contraindicated in patients with peptic ulcer disease or systemic anticoagulation; side effects include gastropathy, nephropathy, liver dysfunction, central nervous system dysfunction and reversible platelet dysfunction; may cause fluid overload in patients with congestive heart failure
Naproxen (Naprosyn)	500 mg two times daily	
Ibuprofen (Motrin)	800 mg four times daily	
Sulindac (Clinoril)	200 mg two times daily	
Ketoprofen (Orudis)	75 mg four times daily	

Corticosteroids		
Oral	Prednisone, 0.5 mg per kg on day 1, taper by 5.0 mg each day thereafter	Fluid retention; impaired wound healing
Intramuscular	Triamcinolone acetonide (Kenalog), 60 mg intramuscularly, repeat in 24 hours if necessary	May require repeat injections; risk of soft tissue atrophy
Intra-articular	Large joints: 10 to 40 mg Small joints: 5 to 20 mg	Preferable route for monoarticular involvement
ACTH	40 to 80 IU intramuscularly; repeat every 8 hours as necessary	Repeat injections are commonly needed; requires intact pituitary-adrenal axis; stimulation of mineralocorticoid release may cause volume overload
Colchicine	0.5 to 0.6 mg PO every hour until relief or side effects occur, or until a maximum dosage of 6 mg is reached	Dose-dependent gastrointestinal side effects; improper intravenous dosing has caused bone marrow suppression, renal failure and death

2. **Corticosteroids**
   a. **Intra-articular, intravenous, intramuscular or oral corticosteroids** are effective in acute gout. In cases where one or two accessible joints are involved, intra-articular injection of corticosteroid can be used.
   b. **Intramuscular triamcinolone acetonide** (60 mg) is as effective as indomethacin in relieving acute gouty arthritis. Triamcinolone acetonide is especially useful in patients with contraindications to NSAIDs.
   c. **Oral prednisone** is an option when repeat dosing is anticipated. Prednisone, 0.5 mg per kg of prednisone on day 1 and tapered by 5 mg each day is very effective.

3. **Colchicine** is effective in treating acute gout; however, 80 percent of patients experience gastrointestinal side effects, including nausea, vomiting and diarrhea. Intravenous colchicine is available but is highly toxic.

C. **Treatment of intercritical gout**
   1. Prophylactic colchicine (from 0.6 mg to 1.2 mg) should be administered at the same time urate-lowering drug therapy is initiate. Colchicine should be used for prophylaxis only with concurrent use of urate-lowering agents. Colchicine is used for prophylaxis until the serum urate concentration is at the desired level and the patient has been free from acute gouty attacks for three to six months.
   2. **Urate-lowering agents**
      a. After the acute gouty attack is treated and prophylactic therapy is initiated, sources of hyperuricemia should be eliminated in hopes of lowering the serum urate level without the use of medication.

b. Medications that may aggravate the patient's condition (eg, diuretics) should be discontinued; purine-rich foods, alcohol consumption should be curtailed, and the patient should gradually lose weight, if obese.

Purine Content of Foods and Beverages

High
Best to avoid: Liver, kidney, anchovies, sardines, herring, mussels, bacon, codfish, scallops, trout, haddock, veal, venison, turkey, alcoholic beverages
Moderate
May eat occasionally: Asparagus, beef, bouillon, chicken, crab, duck, ham, kidney beans, lentils, lima beans, mushrooms, lobster, oysters, pork, shrimp, spinach

3. **24-hour urine uric acid excretion measurement** is essential to identify the most appropriate urate-lowering medication and to check for significant preexisting renal insufficiency.
   a. Uricosuric agents should be used in most patients with gout because most are "underexcretors" of uric acid.
   b. Inhibitors of uric acid synthesis are more toxic and should be reserved for use in "overproducers" of urate (urine excretion >800 mg in 24 hours).
   c. Urate-lowering therapy should not be initiated until the acute attack has resolved, since they may exacerbate the attack.

Urate-Lowering Drugs for the Treatment of Gout and Hyperuricemia

Drug	Dosage	Indications	Side effects/comments
Probene-cid (Bene-mid)	Begin with 250 mg twice daily, gradually titrating upward until the serum urate level is <6 mg per dL; maximum: 3 g per day	Recurrent gout may be combined with allopurinol in resistant hyperuricemia	Uricosuric agent; creatinine clearance must be >60 mL per minute; therapeutic effect reversed by aspirin therapy; avoid concurrent daily aspirin use; contraindicated in urolithiasis; may precipitate gouty attack at start of therapy; rash or gastrointestinal side effects may occur
Allopurinol (Zyloprim)	Begin with 50 to 100 mg daily, gradually titrating upward until the serum urate level is <6 mg per dL; typical dosage: 200 to 300 mg daily	Chronic gouty arthritis; secondary hyperuricemia related to the use of cytolytics in the treatment of hematologic malignancies; gout complicated by renal disease or renal calculi	Inhibits uric acid synthesis; side effects include rash, gastrointestinal symptoms, headache, urticaria and interstitial nephritis; rare, potentially fatal hypersensitivity syndrome

4. **Probenecid (Benemid)** is the most frequently used uricosuric medication. Candidates for probenecid therapy must have hyperuricemia attributed to undersecretion of urate (ie, <800 mg in 24 hours), a creatinine clearance of >60 mL/minute and no history of nephrolithiasis. Probenecid should be initiated at a dosage of 250 mg twice daily and increased as needed, up to 3 g per day, to achieve a serum urate level of less than 6 mg per dL. Side effects include precipitation of an acute gouty attack, renal calculi, and gastrointestinal problems.
5. **Allopurinol (Zyloprim)** is an inhibitor of uric acid synthesis. Allopurinol is initiated at a dosage of 100 mg per day and increased in increments of 50 to 100 mg per day every two weeks until the urate level is <6 mg per dL. Side effects include rash, gastrointestinal problems, headache, urticaria and interstitial nephritis. A hypersensitivity syndrome associated with fever, bone marrow suppression, hepatic toxicity, renal failure and a systemic hypersensitivity vasculitis is rare.

References: See page 195.

Rheumatoid Arthritis

Rheumatoid arthritis (RA) has a prevalence of 0.5-1.0%, and it affects women more often than men. RA tends to develop during early or middle adulthood (between the ages of 20 and 50 years), but it can also begin in childhood or old age. It has only a slight tendency to run in families. RA is a chronic illness, with a course extending over 20 years or more. Nearly 50% of patients with RA may become work disabled after 10 years.

I. **Pathogenesis**. RA is an autoimmune disease, although a virus may trigger the chronic rheumatoid process in vulnerable individuals. This process causes the immune system to attack the synovium of various joints, leading to synovitis. Synovial inflammation accounts for the typical pain warmth, and swelling of the involved joints.

II. **Clinical manifestations**
A. RA is a chronic, symmetric polyarthritis. The polyarthritis is often deforming. About 80% of patients describe a slowly progressive onset over weeks or months. RA may wax and wane, and it may range in intensity from bouts of explosive systemic illness to periods of spontaneous remissions.

B. **Inflammatory features**
1. The joints in RA are swollen, tender, slightly warm, and stiff. Synovial fluid shows active inflammation: The fluid is cloudy and has an increased number of inflammatory white blood cells.
2. Patients with RA usually have profound and prolonged morning stiffness. Fatigue, anemia of chronic disease, and severe constitutional illness (eg, fever, vasculitis, pericarditis, myocarditis, Felty's syndrome) are common.

C. **Joint involvement.** RA may begin in one or two joints, but it almost invariably progresses to affect 20 or more. In some cases, joint involvement is nearly symmetric, affecting the same finger joints on each hand. Initially, the disease typically involves the metacarpophalangeal, proximal interphalangeal, wrist, and metatarsophalangeal joints, either alone or in combination with others. It can then affect virtually any other joint.

D. **Proliferative/erosive features.** The inflamed synovial tissue evolves into a thickened, boggy mass known as a pannus. Pannus can eat through joint cartilage and into adjacent bone, causing radiologically visible erosions.

E. **Joint deformity.** Deformities of RA are more likely to be the result of damage to the soft tissues and supporting structures of the joint -- ligaments, tendons, and joint capsule.

III. **Diagnosis**
A. RA is a clinical diagnosis. The presence of arthritis excludes the many forms

of soft tissue rheumatism (eg, tendinitis, bursitis). The degree of inflammation excludes osteoarthritis and traumatic arthritis. Polyarticular involvement of the appropriate joints makes the spondyloarthropathies unlikely.

B. The pannus is often palpable as a rubbery mass of tissue around a joint. Finding pannus on examination argues strongly against many other forms of polyarthritis, such as that associated with systemic lupus erythematosus.

C. Laboratory tests

1. The rheumatoid factor assay helps to confirm the diagnosis of RA. Rheumatoid factor serves as a marker for RA, but it is not reliable because 1-2% of the normal population have low levels of rheumatoid factor. Chronic infections, other inflammatory conditions and malignancies may trigger formation of rheumatoid factor. Conversely, 15% of patients with RA are seronegative for rheumatoid factor.

2. A positive rheumatoid factor result supports the diagnosis of RA, but a negative test result does not exclude it.

D. Radiography. Typical erosions around joint margins help confirm the diagnosis of RA. Erosions represent relatively late-stage disease.

IV. Treatment of rheumatoid arthritis

A. Disease-modifying antirheumatic drugs

1. Virtually all patients should start taking a disease-modifying antirheumatic drug (DMARDs) as soon as the diagnosis of RA is made. Treatment should continue for the duration of the disease.

2. The early and aggressive use of these agents reduces acute symptoms and decreases disability over the long term. These drugs are no more toxic than high-dose NSAIDs.

3. **Methotrexate** is the treatment of choice because of demonstrated efficacy and long-term tolerability. Therapy should begin with 7.5 mg weekly and increasing at 1- or 2-month intervals until peak efficacy is achieved. Methotrexate is relatively contraindicated with a history of hepatitis or alcoholism. Side effects include anorexia, nausea, vomiting, abdominal cramps, elevated liver enzyme levels, myelosuppression (rare), pulmonary toxicity, hepatic fibrosis, hypersensitivity pneumonitis. Users must be closely monitored for hepatic toxicity.

4. **Hydroxychloroquine (Plaquenil)**, 200-400 mg PO qd, is recommended for patients with mild disease. This drug works slowly but has few side effects. Retinal damage is avoidable if vision is monitored every 6 or 12 months and the drug is stopped when signs of retinal toxicity appear.

B. Etanercept (Enbrel). After twice-weekly subcutaneous injections of etanercept (recombinant human tumor necrosis factor receptor), 25 mg, at 3 months, 62% improve. Etanercept is well tolerated and is an indicated for use alone or with methotrexate for patients with active disease that is refractory to methotrexate.

C. Infliximab (Remicade) is given intravenously for use in refractory disease. Infliximab is an anti-tumor necrosis factor monoclonal antibody. Infliximab is given intravenously in dosages of 3 or 10 mg/kg, repeated at about four-to 12-week intervals.

D. Leflunomide (Arava), which inhibits pyrimidine synthesis, is an oral drug considered as a possible alternative to methotrexate. The dosage is 100 mg PO daily for three days followed by a maintenance dosage of 10 to 20 mg daily. Leflunomide improves rheumatic arthritis but offers no clear advantages over methotrexate.

E. Nonsteroidal antiinflammatory drugs. Most patients will gain short-term symptomatic relief from treatment with NSAIDs. These drugs are generally equivalent in efficacy. NSAIDs can cause peptic ulcer disease and renal insufficiency.

F. Corticosteroids . These drugs may relieve the symptoms of RA, but they are potentially dangerous, with many long-term side effects. They should be reserved for severe systemic disease.

G. **Physical/occupational therapy.** Patients with early hand or joint dysfunction or deformity should undergo physical and occupational therapy assessments for splints, assistive devices, and joint protection.

References: See page 195.

Dermatologic Disorders

Acne Vulgaris

In adolescence, acne affects more boys than girls, and boys tend to have more severe involvement.

I. **Clinical Manifestations**
   A. Acne comedones are usually found on the forehead and upper cheeks of adolescents. Comedones may progress to inflammatory lesions on the lower cheeks, chin, chest, upper back, and shoulders.
   B. In females, the possibility of androgenic disorders such as polycystic ovarian disease and Cushing's syndrome should be considered. The patient should be asked about menstrual irregularities and should be examined for hirsutism.
   C. Acne will often subside during the late teens. However, 20-50% of women seeking acne treatment are in their 20s, and a considerable number have persistent acne into the 30s, 40s, and even 50s.

II. **Non-pharmacologic therapy for acne**
   A. **Diet.** Patients should be advised to eat a well-balanced diet and to avoid foods which consistently result in acne flare-ups.
   B. **Cleanliness.** Development of acne is not related to dirt. Excessive scrubbing may worsen the condition. Patients should be encouraged to wash affected areas with any standard soap once or twice a day and after strenuous physical activities.
   C. **Medications that worsen acne** include oral contraceptives, corticosteroids, anabolic steroids, phenytoin, lithium, and isoniazid.

III. **Pharmacologic therapy**
   A. **Treatment of comedonal acne**
      1. Mild noninflammatory acne can be treated with topical antibacterial agents such as benzoyl peroxide or comedolytic agents such as tretinoin (Retin-A). The combination of benzoyl peroxide in the morning and tretinoin at night is effective.
      2. **Benzoyl peroxide**
         a. Benzoyl peroxide is first-line therapy for mild acne. It is available over-the-counter. The liquids and creams (Benoxyl) are less irritating and are useful for dry skin. The gel (Benzagel, Persa-Gel) is more irritating but more effective for oily skin. Mild redness and scaling occurs during the first week. It may irritate the skin, bleach the clothes, and inactivate simultaneously applied tretinoin and other anti-acne products.
         b. The 2.5% strength is less irritating than higher strengths and equally effective. Apply in the morning and evening after washing [2.5, 5-10% gel, 5-10% cream or lotion].
      3. **Tretinoin (Retin A)**
         a. Prescription retinoids remain the premier agents for both inflammatory and noninflammatory acne. Tretinoin loosens and removes comedones. The agent is available in six different strengths and formulations: a cream (0.025%, 0.05%, 0.1%), a gel (0.01%, 0.025%), and liquid (0.05%).
         b. Fair-skinned patients may begin by applying the 0.025% cream shortly after washing nightly. The quantity of tretinoin applied may be gradually increased as tolerated, and twice-daily applications may be appropriate. The cream is best for dry skin; the gel is best for oily skin.
         c. It should be applied once a day at bedtime after washing.
         d. Retin-A cream (0.025, 0.05, 0.1%) [20, 45 g]; Retin-A gel (0.01,

0.025%) [15, 45 g]; or Retin-A liquid (0.05%) [28 mL].

    e. Mild redness and peeling is common. Excessive sun exposure should be avoided, and sunscreen and protective clothing should be used.

4. **Adapalene (Differin)** is also a topical retinoid, available as a 0.1% gel. It functions in a manner similar to that of tretinoin. Adapalene works slightly better and faster and causes less irritation than tretinoin. Apply once a day to affected areas after washing qhs.

5. **Azelaic acid cream (Azelex)** is indicated for the treatment of acne in patients who cannot tolerate topical tretinoin. Azelaic acid is as effective as tretinoin but with less drying side effects. The 20% cream is applied bid [30 gm].

B. Treatment of pustular acne

1. Moderate or severe inflammatory acne requires oral antibiotics in addition to topical therapy. Side effects of oral antibiotics include gastrointestinal distress and vaginal candidiasis.

2. **Tetracycline**
   a. Tetracycline is an effective and low cost oral antibiotic. Starting dosage is 250 mg qid or 500 mg bid, 1 hour before or 2 hours after meals; after 1-2 months reduce to 250 mg PO qd.
   b. Antacids or dairy products can interfere with absorption; can cause dental discoloration; contraindicated in pregnancy or in children <12 years; photosensitizing.

3. **Minocycline (Minocin).** Highly effective because of lipid solubility and good absorption with food. The usual starting dose is 50 mg bid or 100 mg qd [50,100 mg].

4. **Doxycycline.** Less expensive than minocycline and is very effective. 100 mg once daily; photosensitivity, gastrointestinal distress may occur.

5. **Erythromycin.** Starting dosage is 250 mg qid or 500 mg bid. Propionibacterium acnes bacteria are more resistant to erythromycin than tetracycline; gastrointestinal side effects.

6. **Topical Antibiotics.** Propionibacterium acnes is often resistant to topical antibiotics. Clindamycin is available in 1% solution, lotion or gel (Cleocin-T) for bid application.

7. **Hormone therapy**
   a. In women desiring birth control, an oral contraceptive may mitigate the inflammatory component of acne.
   b. The newer progestins (desogestrel, norgestimate, gestodene) offer exceptional benefits. Ortho Tri-Cyclen and Ortho-Cyclen have an approved indication for moderate acne.
   c. The aldosterone antagonist spironolactone (Aldactone) may provide significant relief for women with hormonal imbalances. At low doses (50 mg/day) it may reduce premenstrual flares.

8. **Isotretinoin (Accutane)**
   a. Isotretinoin is the most potent agent available for treating acne. It decreases sebum production and reverses abnormal epithelial desquamation. Usage is restricted to acne that has not responded to other agents.
   b. **Teratogenicity.** Isotretinoin has the potential to cause severe fetal malformations; therefore, pregnancy must be excluded and contraception is mandatory.
   c. **Initial dose.** 0.5-1.0 mg/kg, or 40-80 mg/day [10,20,40 mg]. Response rate is 90%.

References: See page 195.

Atopic Dermatitis

Eczema includes atopic dermatitis, irritant dermatitis (due to water, detergents, chemicals, heat), and allergic contact dermatitis. The lifetime incidence of atopic dermatitis is 15-20%, with an equal distribution between the sexes.

I. **Atopic Dermatitis**
   A. Atopic dermatitis usually first appears in infants 2-6 months of age. Infants and children have rashes on the shoulders, chest, abdomen, and back. Infants usually also have a rash on the face, scalp and around the ears. Children older than 18 months old tend to have rashes on the neck and antecubital and popliteal fossae.
   B. Atopic dermatitis usually resolves by puberty, but it sometimes recurs at times of stress. In adults it may appear as recalcitrant hand eczema or as a localized dermatitis.
   C. Acute lesions of atopic eczema are itchy, red, edematous papules and small vesicles which may progress to weeping and crusting lesions. Chronic rubbing and scratching may cause lichenification and hyperpigmentation.
   D. The classic triad of atopy consists of asthma, allergic rhinitis, and atopic dermatitis . Atopic dermatitis is associated with a personal or family history of atopy.

Precipitating Factors and Activities in Atopic Dermatitis	
Moisture-related	Excessive bathing, excessive hand washing, excessive lip licking, excessive sweating, extended showers or baths, repeated contact with water (eg, work-related), swimming, occlusive clothing and footwear
Contact-related	Overuse of soap, bubble-bath, cosmetics, deodorants, detergents, solvents, tight clothing, rough fabrics, wool or mohair
Temperature-related	Exposure to excessively warm environment, high humidity, overdressing, hot showers or baths, heating pad
Emotional	Anger, anxiety, depression, stress
Infective	Bacteria, fungi, viruses
Inhalational	Animal dander, cigarette smoke, dust, perfume

II. **Treatment of atopic dermatitis**
   A. **Moisture**
      1. Avoidance of excessive bathing, hand washing, and lip licking should be recommended.
      2. Showers or baths should be limited to no more than 5 minutes. After bathing, patients should apply a moisturizer (Aquaphor, Eucerin, Lubriderm, petrolatum) to noninflamed skin,.
   B. **Contact with irritants**
      1. Overuse of soap should be discouraged. Use of nonirritating soaps (eg,

Dove, Ivory, Neutrogena) should be limited to the axilla, groin, hands, and feet.

2. Infants often have bright red exudative atopic dermatitis (slobber dermatitis) on the cheeks, resulting from drooling. Protection with zinc oxide ointment and a corticosteroid will usually bring improvement.

C. **Topical corticosteroids**

1. Corticosteroid ointments maintain skin hydration and maximize penetration. Corticosteroid creams may sting when applied to acute lesions.

2. Mid- and low-potency topical corticosteroids are used twice-daily for chronic, atopic dermatitis. High-potency steroids may be used for flare-ups, but the potency should be tapered after the dermatitis is controlled.

3. Use of higher potency agents on the face, genitalia and skin-folds may cause epidermal atrophy ("stretch marks"), rebound erythema, and susceptibility to bruising. Only hydrocortisone or low-potency, non-fluorinated steroids should be used in these areas.

Commonly Used Topical Corticosteroids	
Preparation	Size
Low Potency Agents	
Hydrocortisone ointment, cream, 1, 2.5% (Hytone)	30 g
Mild Potency Agents	
Alclometasone dipropionate cream, ointment, 0.05% (Aclovate)	60 g
Triamcinolone acetonide cream, 0.1% (Aristocort)	60 g
Desonide ointment, 0.05% (DesOwen)	60 g
Fluocinolone acetonide cream, 0.01% (Synalar)	60 g
Medium Potency Agents	
Triamcinolone acetonide ointment (Aristocort A), 0.1%	60 g
Betamethasone dipropionate cream (Diprosone), 0.05%	45 g
Triamcinolone acetonide cream, ointment, 0.1% (Kenalog)	60 g
Mometasone cream 0.1% (Elocon)	45 g
Fluocinolone acetonide ointment, 0.025% (Synalar)	60 g
Hydrocortisone butyrate 0.1% cream, ointment (Locoid)	45 g
Betamethasone valerate cream, 0.1% (Valisone)	45 g
Hydrocortisone valerate cream, ointment, 0.2% (Westcort)	60 g

Preparation	Size
High Potency Agents	
Amcinonide ointment, 0.1% (Cyclocort)	60 g
Betamethasone dipropionate ointment (Diprosone) 0.05%	45 g
Fluocinonide cream, ointment, 0.05% (Lidex)	60 g

4. **Allergic reactions to topical corticosteroids** may sometime occur. Allergic reactions to mometasone (Elocon) are rare.
D. **Antihistamines**, such as diphenhydramine or hydroxyzine (Atarax), are somewhat useful for pruritus and are sedating. Nonsedating antihistamines, such as loratadine (Claritin) and fexofenadine (Allegra), are helpful.
E. **Systemic Steroids**
   1. Systemic corticosteroids are reserved for severe, widespread reactions to poison ivy, or for severe involvement of the hands, face, or genitals.
   2. Prednisone, 1-2 mg/kg, is given PO and tapered over 10-18 days. For patients who are at risk for complications of fluid retention due to the mineralocorticoid effects of prednisone, dexamethasone (Decadron), 0.75 mg/kg PO, is used.

References: See page 195.

Common Skin Diseases

I. **Alopecia Areata**
   A. Alopecia areata is characterized by asymptomatic, noninflammatory, non-scarring areas of complete hair loss, most commonly involving the scalp, but the disorder may involve any area of hair-bearing skin.
   B. Auto-antibodies to hair follicles is the most likely cause. Emotional stress is sometimes a precipitating factor. The younger the patient and the more widespread the disease, and the poorer the prognosis.
   C. Regrowth of hair after the first attack takes place in 6 months in 30% of cases, with 50% regrowing within 1 year, and 80% regrowing within 5 years. Ten to 30% of patients will not regrow hair; 5% progress to total hair loss.
   D. Lesions are well defined, single or multiple, round or oval areas of total hair loss. Typical "exclamation point" hairs (hairs 3-10 mm in size with a tapered, less pigmented proximal shaft) are seen at the margins.
   E. **Differential diagnosis:** Tinea capitis, trichotillomania, secondary syphilis, and lupus erythematosus.
   F. A VDRL or RPR test for syphilis should be obtained. A CBC, SMAC, sedimentary rate, thyroid function tests, antinuclear antibody should be done to screen for pernicious anemia, chronic active hepatitis, thyroid disease, lupus erythematosus, and Addison's disease.
   G. **Therapy.** Topical steroids, intralesional steroids, and topical minoxidil may be somewhat effective.

II. **Scabies**
   A. Scabies is an extremely pruritic eruption usually accentuated in the groin, axillae, navel, breasts and finger webs, with sparing the head.
   B. Scabies is spread by skin to skin contact. The diagnosis is established by finding the mite, ova, or feces in scrapings of the skin, usually of the finger webs or genitalia.
   C. Treatment of choice for nonpregnant adults and children is lindane (Kwell),

applied for 8-12 hours, then washed off.

    D. Elimite, a 5% permethrin cream, is more effective but more expensive than lindane (Kwell).

    E. Treatment should be given to all members of an infected household simultaneously. Clothing and sheets must be washed on the day of treatment.

III. Acne Rosacea

    A. This condition commonly presents in fair-skinned individuals and is characterized by papules, erythema, and telangiectasias.

    B. Initial treatment consists of doxycycline or tetracycline. Once there has been some clearing, topical metronidazole gel (Metro-gel) can prevent remission. Sunblock should be used because sunlight can exacerbate the condition.

IV. Seborrheic Dermatitis

    A. Seborrheic dermatitis is often called cradle cap, dandruff, or seborrhea. It has a high prevalence in infancy and then is not common until after puberty. Predilection is for the face, retroauricular region, and upper trunk.

    B. Clinical findings

        1. Infants present with adherent, waxy, scaly lesions on the scalp vertex also known as "cradle cap."

        2. In adults, the eruption is bilaterally symmetrical, affecting the scalp with patchy or diffuse, waxy yellow, greasy scaling on the forehead, retroauricular region, auditory meatus, eyebrows, cheeks, and nasolabial folds.

        3. Trunk areas affected include the presternal, interscapular regions, the umbilicus, intertriginous surfaces of the axilla, inframammary regions, groin, and anogenital crease.

        4. Pruritus is mild, and bacterial infection is indicated by vesiculation and oozing.

    C. Treatment

        1. Scalp. Selenium sulfide or tar shampoos are useful. Topical corticosteroid lotions are used for difficult lesions.

        2. Face, neck, and intertriginous regions. Hydrocortisone 1 or 2 ½%.

        3. Trunk. Fluorinated steroids can be used if severe lesions are present.

V. Drug Eruptions

    A. Drug eruptions may be type I, type II, type III, or type IV immunologic reactions. Cutaneous drug reactions may start within 7 days of initiation of the drug or within 4-7 days after the offending drug has been stopped.

    B. The cutaneous lesions usually become more severe and widespread over the following several days to 1 week and then clear over the next 7-14 days.

    C. Lesions most often start first and clear first from the head and upper extremities to the trunk and lower legs. Palms, soles, and mucous membranes may be involved.

    D. Most drug reactions appear as a typical maculopapular drug reaction. Tetracycline is associated with a fixed drug eruption; thiazide diuretics have a tendency for photosensitivity eruptions.

    E. Treatment of drug eruptions

        1. Oral antihistamines are very useful. Diphenhydramine (Benadryl), 25-50 mg q4-6h.

        2. Soothing, tepid water baths in Aveeno or corn starch or cool compresses are useful.

        3. Severe signs and symptoms. A 2-week course of systemic steroids (prednisone starting at 60 mg/day and then tapering) will usually stop the symptoms and prevent further progression of the eruption.

    F. Erythema Multiforme

        1. Erythema multiforme presents as dull red macules or papules on the back of hands, palms, wrists, feet, elbows and knees. The periphery is red and the center becomes blue or darker red, hence the characteristic target or iris lesion.

2. It is most commonly a drug reaction caused by sulfa medications or phenytoin (Dilantin). It is also seen as a reaction to herpes simplex virus infections, mycoplasma, and Hepatitis B.

3. Erythema multiforme major or Steven's Johnson syndrome is diagnosed when mucous membrane or eye involvement is present.

4. Prednisone 30-60 mg/day is often given with a 2-4 week taper.

5. For HSV-driven erythema multiforme, acyclovir may be helpful. Ophthalmologic consultation is obtained for ocular involvement.

VI. Paronychias

A. Chronic infections around the edge of the nail, paronychias, are caused almost universally to Candida albicans. Moisture predisposes to Candida.

B. Acute perionychia presents as tender, red, swollen areas of the nail fold, but not the nail itself. Pus may be seen through the nail plate or at the paronychial fold. The most common causative bacteria are staphylococci, beta-hemolytic streptococci, and gram-negative enteric bacteria. Predisposing factors to perionychia include minor trauma and splinters under the nail.

C. **Diagnosis of paronychial lesions.** Chronic lesions are usually caused by Candida and may be diagnosed by KOH prep or by fungal culture. Acute lesions are usually bacterial and may be cultured for bacteria.

D. **Treatment of chronic candida paronychia**
1. Stop all wet work and apply clotrimazole (Lotrimin) 1% solution tid.
2. Resistant cases can be treated with a 3-6 week oral course of fluconazole (Diflucan), 100 mg PO daily, or itraconazole (Sporanox), 200-400 mg PO daily.

E. **Treatment of acute bacterial paronychia** consists of dicloxacillin 500 mg PO qid, cephalexin (Keflex) 500 mg PO qid, cefadroxil (Duricef) 500 mg PO bid, or erythromycin 500 mg PO qid. If redness and swelling do not resolve, and a pocket of pus remains, drainage is indicated.

VII. Pityriasis Versicolor

A. Pityriasis versicolor (tinea versicolor) most commonly presents as small perifollicular, scaly, hypopigmented or hyperpigmented patches on the upper trunk in young adults. The perifollicular patches expand over time and become confluent.

B. In tinea versicolor, fungus does not grow in standard fungal culture media (eg, Sabouraud's dextrose), but KOH examination shows the abundant "spaghetti and meatballs" pattern of short hyphae and round spores. Pityrosporon ovale is part of the normal flora of skin in amounts that are not detectable on KOH examination. It is a yeast infection, and it is not a dermatophyte infection.

C. Effective topical treatment consists of selenium sulfide 2.5% lotion (Exsel, Selsun) applied overnight once a week for 3 weeks. Topical antifungal creams may also be used.
1. Miconazole (Micatin); apply to affected areas bid; 2% cream.
2. Clotrimazole (Lotrimin), apply to affected area bid for up to 4 wk; cream: 1% [15, 30, 45, 90 gm],1% lotion.
3. Ketoconazole (Nizoral) apply to affected area(s) qd-bid; 2% cream.

D. Effective systemic treatment consists of fluconazole (Diflucan), 400 mg, or ketoconazole (Nizoral), 400 mg, given as a single dose.

E. Relapses are very common. Prophylactic therapy, once weekly to monthly, with topical or oral agents should be encouraged if relapses occur.

VIII. Pityriasis Rosea

A. Pityriasis rosea is an acute inflammatory dermatitis characterized by self-limited lesions distributed on the trunk and extremities. A viral cause is hypothesized. It is most common between the ages of 10 and 35.

B. **Clinical manifestations**
1. The initial lesion, called the "herald patch", can appear anywhere on the body, and is 2-6 cm in size, and begins a few days to several weeks

before the generalized eruption. The hands, face, and feet are usually spared.

2. The lesions are oval, and the long axes follow the lines of cleavage. Lesions are 2 cm or less, pink, tan, or light brown. The borders of the lesions have a loose rim of scales, peeling peripherally, called the "collarette." Pruritus is usually minimal.

C. Differential Diagnosis. Secondary syphilis (always check a VDRL for atypical rashes), drug eruptions, viral exanthems, acute papular psoriasis, tinea corporis.

D. Treatment. Topical antipruritic emollients (Caladryl) relieve itching. Ultraviolet therapy may be used within the first week. The disease usually resolves in 2-14 weeks and recurrences are unusual.

References: See page 195.

Tinea Infections

About 10-20 percent of persons acquire a dermatophyte infection during their lifetime. Dermatophyte infections are classified according to the affected body site, such as tinea capitis (scalp), tinea barbae (beard area), tinea corporis (skin other than bearded area, scalp, groin, hands or feet), tinea cruris (groin, perineum and perineal areas), tinea pedis (feet), tinea manuum (hands) and tinea unguium (nails).

I. Diagnosis

A. Microscopy. Material is scraped from an active area of the lesion, placed in a drop of potassium hydroxide solution, and examined under a microscope.

B. Microscopy is positive if hyphae are identified in fungal infections and if pseudohyphae or yeast forms are seen in Candida or Pityrosporum infections. A positive examination is sufficient to warrant starting treatment.

C. Cultures are not routinely performed in suspected tinea infections. However, cultures should be obtained when long-term oral drug therapy is being considered, the patient has a recalcitrant infection, or the diagnosis is in doubt.

II. Tinea capitis

A. Tinea capitis primarily affects school-aged children, appearing as one or more round patches of alopecia. Hair shafts broken off at the scalp may appear as black dots. Sometimes tinea capitis appears as non-specific dandruff, or gray patches of hair, or areas of scales, pustules and erythema. A localized, boggy, indurated granuloma called a "kerion" may develop.

B. Tinea capitis should be treated with oral therapy. Griseofulvin (Fulvicin PG, Gris-PEG, Grisactin Ultra). Itraconazole (Sporanox) and terbinafine (Lamisil) are effective options.

III. Tinea barbae. Tinea barbae affects the beard area of men who work with animals. It is often accompanied by bacterial folliculitis and inflammation secondary to ingrown hairs. Oral therapy with griseofulvin, itraconazole (Sporanox) or terbinafine (Lamisil) is preferred over topical therapy because the involved hair follicles do not respond well to topical therapy.

IV. Tinea corporis

A. Tinea corporis ("ringworm") often affects children and adults who live in hot, humid climates. The classic presentation of this infection is a lesion with central clearing surrounded by an advancing, red, scaly, elevated border.

B. Since tinea corporis can be asymptomatic, it can spread rapidly among children in day-care settings. Unless only one or two lesions are present, tinea corporis should be treated orally. Terbinafine and itraconazole are equally effective in treating tinea corporis. These agents have a better cure rate than griseofulvin. An alternative is fluconazole (Diflucan), which is given orally once a week for up to four consecutive weeks.

V. Tinea cruris

A. Tinea cruris ("jock itch") usually involves the medial aspect of the upper thighs (groin). Unlike yeast infections, tinea cruris generally does not involve the scrotum or the penis. This dermatophyte infection occurs more often in men than in women and rarely affects children. Erythematous, pruritic plaques often develop bilaterally.

B. Topical therapy is sufficient in most patients with tinea cruris. If the infection spreads to the lower thighs or buttocks, oral therapy with itraconazole or terbinafine is recommended.

VI. Tinea pedis

A. Tinea pedis ("athlete's foot") is the most common dermatophyte infection. Tinea pedis infection is usually related to sweating, warmth, and oclusive footwear. The infection often presents as white, macerated areas in the third or fourth toe webs or as chronic dry, scaly hyperkeratosis of the soles and heels.

B. Occasionally, tinea pedis may produce acute, highly inflamed, sterile vesicles at distant sites (arms, chest, sides of fingers). Referred to as the "dermatophytid" or "id" reaction, these vesicles probably represent an immunologic response to the fungus; they subside when the primary infection is controlled. The "id" reaction can be the only manifestation of an asymptomatic web space infection.

C. Tinea pedis is often treated with topical therapy. Oral itraconazole and terbinafine are more efficacious in the treatment of hyperkeratotic tinea pedis. Once-weekly dosing with fluconazole is another option, especially in noncompliant patients.

VII. Tinea manuum is a fungal infection of the hands. Tinea manuum presents with erythema and mild scaling on the dorsal aspect of the hands or as a chronic, dry, scaly hyperkeratosis of the palms. When the palms are infected, the feet are also commonly infected. Treatment options are the same as for tinea pedis.

VIII. Tinea unguium

A. Tinea unguium is a dermatophyte infection of the nails. It is a subset of onychomycosis, which includes dermatophyte, nondermatophyte and yeast infections of the nails. Toenails are involved more frequently than fingernails. Risk factors for this fungal infection include increasing age, diabetes, poor venous and lymphatic drainage, ill-fitting shoes, and sports participation. Involvement of the toenail usually is extremely resistant to treatment and has a tendency to recur. Chemical or surgical avulsion may be helpful in recalcitrant infection.

B. With distal involvement, the affected nail is hyperkeratotic, chalky and dull. The brownish-yellow debris that forms beneath the nail causes the nail to separate from its bed. Coexistent tinea manuum or tinea pedis is common.

C. Tinea unguium requires oral itraconazole or terbinafine. Itraconazole "pulse" therapy (ie, a series of brief medication courses) is recommended for tinea unguium of the fingernails and toenails. Terbinafine pulse therapy may also be effective. Fluconazole may be another alternative.

Topical Treatments for Tinea Pedis, Tinea Cruris and Tinea Corporis

Antifungal agent	Prescription	Cream	Solution or spray	Lotion	Powder	Frequency of application
Imidazoles						
Clotrimazole 1 percent (Lotrimin, Mycelex)		X	X	X		Twice daily
Miconazole 2 percent (Micatin, Monistat-Derm)		X	X	X	X	Twice daily
Econazole 1 percent (Spectazole)	X	X				Once daily
Ketoconazole 2 percent (Nizoral)	X	X	X			Once daily
Oxiconazole 1 percent (Oxistat)	X	X		X		Once daily or twice daily
Allylamines						
Naftifine 1 percent (Naftin)	X	X				Once daily or twice daily
Terbinafine 1 percent (Lamisil)	X	X	X			Once daily or twice daily

Recommended Dosages and Durations of Oral Therapy for Tinea Infections

Antifungal agent	Tinea capitis	Tinea corporis/cruris	Tinea pedis	Tinea unguium Fingernails	Tinea unguium Toenails
Terbinafine (Lamisil)	Adults: 250 mg per day for four to six weeks Children: 3 to 6 mg per kg per day for six weeks	Adults: 250 mg per day for one to four weeks	250 mg per day for two to six weeks	Continuous: 250 mg per day for six weeks Pulse: 500 mg per day for one week on, three weeks off, for a total of two months	Continuous: 250 mg per day for 12 weeks Pulse: 500 mg per day for one week on, three weeks off, for a total of four months
Itraconazole (Sporanox)	Adults: 100 mg per day for six weeks Children: 3 to 5 mg per kg per day for four to six weeks	100 mg per day for two weeks or 200 mg per day for two weeks or 200 mg per day for one to two weeks	100 mg per day for four weeks	Continuous: 200 mg per day for six weeks Pulse: 200 mg twice daily for one week on, three weeks off, for two months	Continuous: 200 mg per day for 12 weeks Pulse: 200 mg twice daily for one week on, three weeks off, for three to four months
Fluconazole (Diflucan)	50 mg per day for three weeks	150 mg weekly for two to four weeks	150 mg weekly for two to six weeks	Not recommended	Not recommended

IX. Treatment selection

A. Topical antifungal preparations

1. Treatment of tinea infections with topical preparations has limited efficacy because of the lengthy duration of treatment and high relapse rates.

2. Ointment preparations soften thickened, hyperkeratotic lesions. Lotions and solutions prevent maceration in intertriginous areas and hairy areas of the body. Cream formulations are beneficial in the treatment of scaling, non-oozing lesions. Powders alone are less effective. However, they are helpful as adjunctive agents for reducing moisture and maceration, and they can prevent fungal infections in intertriginous areas.

B. Oral antifungal agents

1. Oral therapy is often chosen because of its shorter duration and greater compliance. However, oral agents must be used for disease that is extensive, that affects hair and nails, or that does not respond to topical agents.

2. **Terbinafine (Sporanox)** has fewer drug interactions because it minimally affects the cytochrome P_{450} enzyme system. Itraconazole, fluconazole and ketoconazole significantly inhibit this system.

3. **Side effects of fluconazole (Diflucan)** include rash, headache, gastrointestinal disorders and elevated liver function levels. Erythema multiforme may rarely occur.

4. **Side effects of terbinafine (Lamisil)** include skin rashes and gastrointestinal upset. It has also been associated with Stevens-Johnson syndrome, blood dyscrasias, hepatotoxicity and ocular disturbances, as well as elevated liver enzyme levels in 0.5%. Some patients have noted losing their sense of taste for up to six weeks.

5. **Topical corticosteroids** are beneficial in the initial stages of treatment because they suppress the inflammatory response and provide symptomatic relief. Because of the possibility of fungal proliferation, topical corticosteroids should not be used alone in the treatment of tinea infections.

References: See page 195.

Bacterial Infections of the Skin

I. Furuncles and Carbuncles

A. A furuncle, or boil, is an acute perifollicular staphylococcal abscess of the skin and subcutaneous tissue. Lesions appear as an indurated, dull, red nodule with a central purulent core, usually beginning around a hair follicle or a sebaceous gland. Furuncles occur most commonly on the nape, face, buttocks, thighs, perineum, breast, and axillae.

B. A carbuncle is a coalescence of interconnected furuncles that drain through a number of points on the skin surface.

C. The most common cause of furuncles and carbuncles is coagulase-positive S aureus. Cultures should be obtained from all suppurative lesions.

D. Treatment of furuncles and carbuncles

1. Warm compresses and cleansing.

2. Dicloxacillin (Pathocil) 500 mg PO qid for 2 weeks.

3. Manipulation and surgical incision of early lesions should be avoided, because these maneuvers may cause local or systemic extension. However, when the lesions begin to suppurate and become fluctuant, drainage may be performed by "nicking" the lesion with a No. 11 blade.

4. Draining lesions should be covered with topical antibiotics and loose dressings.

II. Superficial Folliculitis
A. Superficial folliculitis is characterized by small dome-shaped pustules at the ostium of hair follicles. It is caused by coagulase-positive S aureus. Multiple or single lesions appear on the scalp, back, and extremities. In children, the scalp is the most common site.

B. Gram stain and bacterial culture supports the diagnosis.

C. **Treatment.** Local cleansing and erythromycin 2% solution applied topically bid to affected areas.

III. Impetigo
A. Impetigo consists of small superficial vesicles, which eventually form pustules and develop a honey-colored crust. A halo of erythema often surrounds the lesions.

B. Impetigo occurs most commonly on exposed surfaces such as the extremities and face, where minor trauma, insect bites, contact dermatitis, or abrasions may have occurred.

C. Gram stain of an early lesion or the base of a crust often reveals gram-positive cocci.

D. **Treatment of impetigo**
1. A combination of systemic and topical therapy is recommended for moderate to severe cases of impetigo for a 7- to 10-day course:
   a. Dicloxacillin 250-500 mg PO qid.
   b. Cephalexin (Keflex) 250-500 mg PO qid.
   c. Erythromycin 250-500 mg PO qid is used in penicillin allergic patients.
2. Mupirocin (Bactroban) is highly effective against staphylococci and Streptococcus pyogenes. Applied bid-tid for 2-3 weeks or until 1 week after lesions heal. Bacitracin (neomycin, polymyxin B) ointment tid may also be used.

E. **Complications**
1. Acute glomerulonephritis is a serious complication of impetigo, with an incidence of 2-5%. It is most commonly seen in children under the age of 6 years old. Treatment of impetigo does not alter the risk of acute glomerulonephritis.
2. Rheumatic fever has not been reported after impetigo.

IV. Cellulitis
A. Cellulitis is a diffuse suppurative bacterial inflammation of the subcutaneous tissue. It is characterized by localized erythema, warmth, and tenderness. Cutaneous erythema is poorly demarcated from uninvolved skin. Cellulitis may be accompanied by malaise, fever, and chills.

B. The most common causes are beta-hemolytic streptococcal and S aureus. Complications include gangrene, metastatic abscesses, and sepsis.

C. **Treatment**
1. Dicloxacillin or cephalexin provide coverage for streptococci and staphylococci. Penicillin may be added to increase activity against streptococci.
2. **Antibiotic Therapy**
   a. Dicloxacillin (Dycill, Pathocil) 40 mg/kg/day in 4 divided doses for 7-12 days; adults: 500 mg qid.
   b. Cephalexin (Keflex) 50 mg/kg/day PO in 4 divided doses for 7-10 days; adults: 500 mg PO qid.
   c. Amoxicillin/clavulanate (Augmentin) 500 mg tid or 875 mg bid for 7-10 days.
   d. Azithromycin (Zithromax) 500 mg on day 1, then 250 mg PO qd for 4 days.
   e. Erythromycin ethylsuccinate 40 mg/kg/day in 3 divided doses for 7-10 days; adults: 250-500 mg qid.

References: See page 195.

Psoriasis

Psoriasis affects about 1 to 3 percent of the population. While patients with extensive and severe disease may require potent oral therapy, less severe psoriasis is typically treated with topical medications. Psoriasis is caused by a shortened epidermal cell cycle, resulting from a primary immunologic disorder that leads to secondary epidermal hyperproliferation.

I. Clinical evaluation
   A. The lesions are elevated and erythematous, with thick, silver scales. Scraping off the scale leaves a bleeding point (Auspitz sign). Lesion have a predilection for the sacral region, over extensor surfaces (elbows, knees, lumbosacral), and scalp. Other lesions may appear at sites of trauma (Koebner's phenomenon), such as an excoriation.
   B. Medications that can trigger the onset of psoriasis include beta-blockers, lithium, nonsteroidal anti-inflammatory agents, and progesterone-containing oral contraceptives.
   C. Mucosal psoriasis consist of circinate, ring-shaped, whitish lesions on the tongue, palate, or buccal mucosa. Onycholysis, or separation of the nail plate from the underlying nail bed is frequently seen, as well as a yellow-brown discoloration underneath the nail, known as an "oil spot."
   D. Psoriatic arthritis occurs in 20-34% of patients with psoriasis. It is characterized by asymmetrical distal oligoarthritis involving small joints; a smaller number of patients have a symmetrical arthritis of the larger joints or a spondyloarthropathy. The arthritis may be mutilating and destructive.

II. Treatment of psoriasis
   A. Corticosteroid therapy
      1. Topical corticosteroids are the most widely used treatment for psoriasis. Corticosteroids have anti-inflammatory, immunosuppressive and antiproliferative properties.
      2. Mid-potency corticosteroids are used for lesions on the torso and extremities, while low-potency corticosteroids are used for areas with delicate skin, such as that on the face, genitals or flexures. These delicate areas are at increased risk for cutaneous atrophy. High-potency corticosteroids are usually reserved for use on recalcitrant plaques or lesions on the palms of the hands and soles of the feet. They should not be used for more than two weeks.

Corticosteroid Potency	
Generic name	Trade name and strength
Superpotent	
Betamethasone dipropionate	Diprolene gel/ointment, 0.05% [45 g]
Diflorasone diacetate	Psorcon ointment, 0.05% [45 g]
Clobetasol propionate	Temovate cream/ointment, 0.05% [45 g]
Halobetasol propionate	Ultravate cream/ointment, 0.05% [45 g]

Generic name	Trade name and strength
Potent	
Amcinonide	Cyclocort ointment, 0.1% [60 g]
Betamethasone dipropionate	Diprosone ointment, 0.05% [45 g]
Desoximetasone	Topicort cream/ointment, 0.25%; gel 0.05% [45 g]
Diflorasone diacetate	Florone ointment, 0.05%; Maxiflor ointment, 0.05% [45 g]
Fluocinonide	Lidex cream/ointment, 0.05% [60 g]
Halcinonide	Halog cream, 0.1% [45 g]
Upper mid-strength	
Betamethasone dipropionate	Diprosone cream, 0.05% [45 g]
Betamethasone valerate	Valisone ointment, 0.1% [45 g]
Diflorasone diacetate	Florone, Maxiflor creams, 0.05%
Mometasone furoate	Elocon ointment, 0.1% [45 g]
Triamcinolone acetonide	Aristocort cream, 0.5% [45 g]
Mid-strength	
Desoximetasone	Topicort LP cream, 0.05% [60 g]
Fluocinolone acetonide	Synalar-HP cream, 0.2%; Synalar ointment, 0.025% [60 g]
Flurandrenolide	Cordran ointment, 0.05% [60 g]
Triamcinolone acetonide	Aristocort, Kenalog ointments, 0.1% [60 g]
Lower mid-strength	
Betamethasone dipropionate	Diprosone lotion, 0.05% [60 g]
Betamethasone valerate	Valisone cream/lotion, 0.1% [45 g]
Fluocinolone acetonide	Synalar cream, 0.025% [45 g]
Flurandrenolide	Cordran cream, 0.05% [45 g]
Hydrocortisone butyrate	Locoid cream, 0.1% [45 g]

Generic name	Trade name and strength
Hydrocortisone valerate	Westcort cream, 0.2% [45 g]
Prednicarbate	Dermatop emollient cream, 0.1%
Triamcinolone acetonide	Kenalog cream/lotion, 0.1% [60 g]
Mild	
Alclometasone dipropionate	Aclovate cream/ointment, 0.05% [60 g]
Triamcinolone acetonide	Aristocort cream, 0.1% [60 g]
Desonide	DesOwen cream, 0.05% [60 g]
Fluocinolone acetonide	Synalar cream/solution, 0.01% [60 g]
Betamethasone valerate	Valisone lotion, 0.1% [45 g]

3. **Ointments** are best for dry, scaly, hyperkeratotic plaques. Lotions and gels are best suited for the scalp; creams can be used on all areas.
4. **Corticosteroid therapy** may cause tachyphylaxis, leading to decreased efficacy with continued use and culminating in an acute flare-up when therapy is terminated. Tachyphylaxis can be minimized by switching to less potent corticosteroids and having them apply the medication less frequently once the lesions have improved. Local side effects include acne and localized hypertrichosis.
5. **Skin atrophy** can also occur and may lead to striae, telangiectasia and purpura. The use of very potent corticosteroids or weaker ones under occlusion may lead to suppression of the pituitary-adrenal axis. Systemic absorption can minimize by limiting use to <40-50 g/week of a potent corticosteroid and not more than 90-100 g/week of a moderately potent corticosteroid.

Topical Agents for Psoriasis

Drug	Advantages	Disadvantages	Comment
Corticosteroids	Easy to use, rapid onset	Tachyphylaxis, atrophy, telangiectasia and adrenal suppression possible	Can be used in combination with calcipotriene (Dovonex) or tazarotene (Tazorac)
Calcipotriene (Dovonex)	Well-tolerated	Expensive, may cause skin irritation	Potential for hypercalcemia with excessive use
Anthralin (Anthra-Derm)	Once-daily administration, well-tolerated	May stain and/or cause skin irritation	Microencapsulated form may be less staining and irritating

Drug	Advantages	Disadvantages	Comment
Tars	Effective with UV light therapy	May cause skin staining, folliculitis, contact allergy; malodorous	Commonly used for psoriasis of the scalp
Tazarotene (Tazorac)		Expensive, may be teratogenic; irritating to uninvolved skin	First topical retinoid indicated by the FDA for treatment of psoriasis

    B. Keratolytics assist in removing scale or hyperkeratosis. Salicylic acid is usually prescribed in concentrations between 2 and 10 percent and should not be applied extensively on the body because salicylism (tinnitus, nausea, vomiting) may result.

    C. Coal tar has antiproliferative and anti-inflammatory actions. It is beneficial when used alone in mild to moderate psoriasis, and is useful in combination with ultraviolet B radiation. The use of coal tar is limited by its unpleasant odor; it can also stain clothing and bedding.

    D. Vitamin D analogs

        1. Calcipotriene (Dovonex), a topical vitamin D analog, is as effective as betamethasone valerate ointment. The short-term response to calcipotriene can be maintained for up to 12 months.

        2. Calcipotriene, applied twice daily, is well tolerated, although the face and groin areas should be avoided since it may cause irritant dermatitis. To avoid hypercalcemia, use should not exceed 100 g/week.

    E. Retinoids

        1. Retinoids mediate cell differentiation and proliferation. Tazarotene (Tazorac) use may lead to an extended response, providing long-term improvement and maintenance therapy.

        2. Local skin irritation and pruritus are frequent side effects. Since tazarotene may be teratogenic; women of child-bearing age should use adequate birth-control measures. A negative pregnancy test should be confirmed within two weeks of initiating treatment.

    F. Phototherapy and systemic therapy

        1. Patients with psoriatic involvement of greater than 10%% of body surface area or with severe, incapacitating, or disfiguring psoriasis are candidates for photochemotherapy or systemic therapy.

        2. **UV light** therapy is effective for psoriatic lesions. Phototherapy with ultraviolet A light and psoralens (PUVA) is effective widespread lesions. Daily sunlight exposure can benefit most patients; however, overexposure can exacerbate the disease.

        3. **Systemic therapies** include methotrexate, etretinate (Tegison), cyclosporine, and hydroxyurea, and these therapies have better than an 80% response rate.

References: See page 195.

Gynecologic Disorders

Management of the Abnormal Pap Smear

There has been a steady decrease in the incidence of cervical cancer with the widespread use of Pap smears. Intraepithelial neoplasia of the cervix usually occurs in young women. A major factor in development of CIN is the human papillomavirus (HPV), which is the most common sexually transmitted disease. Additional epidemiologic factors are the early age of first intercourse, early childbearing, and multiple sexual partners.

I. **Screening for cervical cancer**
   A. Regular Pap smears are recommended for all women who are or have been sexually active and who have a cervix.
   B. Testing should begin when the woman first engages in sexual intercourse. Adolescents whose sexual history is thought to be unreliable should be presumed to be sexually active at age 18.
   C. Pap smears should be performed at least every 1 to 3 years. Testing is usually discontinued after age 65 in women who have had regular normal screening tests. Women who have had a hysterectomy including removal of the cervix for reasons other than cervical cancer or its precursors do not require Pap testing.

II. **Management of minor Pap smear abnormalities**
   A. **Satisfactory, but limited by few (or absent) endocervical cells**
      1. Endocervical cells are absent in up to 10% of Pap smears before menopause and up to 50% postmenopausally.
      2. **Management.** The Pap smear should either be repeated annually or only recall women with previously abnormal Pap smears.
   B. **Unsatisfactory for evaluation**
      1. Repeat Pap smear midcycle in 6-12 weeks.
      2. If atrophic smear, treat with estrogen cream for 6-8 weeks, then repeat Pap smear.
   C. **Benign cellular changes**
      1. **Infection--Candida**. Most cases represent asymptomatic colonization. Treatment is offered for symptomatic cases. The Pap should be repeated at usual interval.
      2. **Infection--Trichomonas**. If wet preparation is positive, treat with metronidazole (Flagyl), then continue annual Pap smears.
      3. **Infection--predominance of coccobacilli consistent with shift in vaginal flora.** This finding implies bacterial vaginosis, but it is a non-specific finding. Diagnosis should be confirmed by findings of a homogeneous vaginal discharge, positive amine test, and clue cells on saline suspension.
      4. **Infection-herpes simplex virus.** Pap smear has poor sensitivity but good specificity for HSV; positive smears usually are caused by asymptomatic infection. The patient should be informed of pregnancy risks and the possibility of transmission. No treatment is necessary, and the Pap should be repeated as for a benign result.
      5. **Inflammation on Pap smear**
         a. **Mild inflammation** on an otherwise normal smear does not need further evaluation.
         b. **Moderate or severe inflammation** should be evaluated with a saline preparation, KOH preparation, and gonorrhea and Chlamydia tests. If the source of infection is found, treatment should be provided, and a repeat Pap smear should be done every 6 to 12 months. If no etiology is found, the Pap smear should be repeated in 6 months.
         c. **Persistent inflammation** may be infrequently the only manifestation

of high-grade squamous intraepithelial lesions (HGSIL) or invasive cancer; therefore, persistent inflammation is an indication for colposcopy.

6. **Atrophy with inflammation** is common in post-menopausal women or in those with estrogen-deficiency states. Atrophy should be treated with vaginal estrogen for 4-6 weeks, then repeat Pap smear.

7. **Hyperkeratosis and parakeratosis**. Parakeratosis is defined as dense nuclei within a keratin layer. When no nuclei are present, the cells are designated hyperkeratotic. Parakeratosis and hyperkeratosis occur as a reaction to physical, chemical, or inflammatory trauma, and it may clinically appear as leukoplakia. Benign-appearing parakeratosis or hyperkeratosis requires only a repeat Pap test in 6 months. When this finding persists, colposcopy is indicated.

III. Management of squamous cell abnormalities

A. Atypical squamous cells of undetermined significance (ASCUS)

1. ASCUS indicates cells with nuclear atypia, but not atypia caused by human papilloma (HPV).

2. With a conservative approach to ASCUS smears, the patient is asked to return every 6 months for a repeat Pap smear. The American College of Obstetricians and Gynecologists (ACOG) advises a colposcopic examination if a patient receives two or more ASCUS reports (repeat Pap smears being obtained every 6 months) or if the patient's compliance is uncertain with the original report.

B. Low-grade squamous intraepithelial lesions (LGSIL)

1. LSIL includes human papilloma virus (HPV) and CIN 1 (or mild dysplasia). Koilocytotic atypia is indicative of HPV.

2. A significant number of LGSIL smears represent processes that will revert spontaneously to normal without therapy. Repeat Pap smears every 4 to 6 months is recommended, with colposcopy being indicated if there is persistence or progression. However, because some women will progress and because of the high rate of false-negative Pap smears, clinicians may perform colposcopy after the initial LGSIL report.

C. High-grade squamous intraepithelial lesion (HSIL).

1. If the Pap smear is consistent with HSIL (or persistent or high-risk LSIL), colposcopy and biopsy should be performed.

   a. If biopsy results are consistent with CIN I, provide careful observation and follow-up.

   b. If biopsy results are consistent with CIN II or III, cryotherapy, laser vaporization, LEEP or cone biopsy should be completed. If biopsy results are consistent with invasive disease, further staging procedures are indicated.

IV. Management of glandular cell abnormalities

A. Endometrial cells on Pap smear.

When a Pap smear is performed during menstruation, endometrial cells may be present. However, endometrial cells on a Pap smear performed during the second half of the menstrual cycle or in a post-menopausal patient may indicate the presence of polyps, hyperplasia, or endometrial adenocarcinoma. An endometrial biopsy should be considered in these women.

B. Atypical glandular cells of undetermined significance (AGUS).

Colposcopically directed biopsy and endocervical curettage is recommended in all women with AGUS smears, and abnormal endometrial cells should be investigated by endometrial biopsy, fractional curettage, or hysteroscopy.

C. Adenocarcinoma.

This diagnosis requires endocervical curettage, cone biopsy, and/or endometrial biopsy.

V. Colposcopically directed biopsy

A. Liberally apply a solution of 3-5% acetic acid to cervix, and inspect cervix for abnormal areas (white epithelium, punctation, mosaic cells, atypical

vessels). Biopsies of any abnormal areas should be obtained under colposcopic visualization. Record location of each biopsy. Monsel solution may be applied to stop bleeding.
   B. **Endocervical curettage** is done routinely during colposcopy, except during pregnancy.
VI. **Treatment based on cervical biopsy findings**
   A. **Benign cellular changes (infection, reactive inflammation).** Treat the infection, and repeat the smear every 4-6 months; after 2 negatives, repeat yearly.
   B. **Squamous intraepithelial lesions**
      1. Women with SIL should be treated on the basis of the histological biopsy diagnosis. Patients with CIN I require no further treatment because the majority of these lesions resolve spontaneously. Patients with CIN II or CIN III require treatment to prevent development of invasive disease.
      2. These lesions are treated with cryotherapy, laser vaporization, or loop electric excision procedure (LEEP).

References: See page 195.

Contraception

One-half of unplanned pregnancies occur among the 10 percent of women who do not use contraception. The remainder of unintended pregnancies result from contraceptive failure.

Advantages and Disadvantages of Various Birth Control Methods		
Method	**Advantages**	**Disadvantages**
Diaphragm	Inexpensive; some protection against STDs other than HIV	Not to be used with oil-based lubricants; latex allergy; urinary tract infections
Cervical cap (Prentif Cavit)	Inexpensive; some protection against STDs other than HIV	Damaged by oil-based lubricants; latex allergy; toxic shock syndrome; decreased efficacy with increased frequency of intercourse; difficult to use
Intrauterine device	Long-term use (up to 10 years)	Increased bleeding, spotting or cramping; risk of ectopic pregnancy with failure; risk of infertility; no protection against HIV and other STDs
Oral combination contraceptive	Decreased menstrual flow and cramping; decreased incidence of pelvic inflammatory disease, ovarian and endometrial cancers, ovarian cyst, ectopic pregnancy, fibrocystic breasts, fibroids, endometriosis and toxic shock syndrome; highly effective	Increased risk of benign hepatic adenomas; mildly increased risk of blood pressure elevation or thromboembolism; no protection against HIV and other STDs; nausea

Method	Advantages	Disadvantages
Progestin-only agent	Compatible with breast-feeding; no estrogenic side effects	Possible amenorrhea; must be taken at the same time every day; no protection against HIV; nausea
Depot-medroxy-progesterone acetate (Depo-Provera)	Decreased or no menstrual flow or cramps; compatible with breast-feeding; highly effective	Delayed return of fertility; irregular bleeding; decreased libido; no protection against HIV; nausea
Levonorgestrel implant (Norplant)	Decreased menstrual flow, cramping and ovulatory pain; no adherence requirements; highly effective	Costly; surgical procedure required for insertion; no protection against HIV
Tubal ligation	Low failure rate; no adherence requirements	Surgery; no protection against HIV and other STDs
Vasectomy	Low failure rate; no adherence requirements; outpatient procedure	Surgical procedure; postoperative infection; no protection against HIV
Condoms (male and female)	Inexpensive; some protection against HIV infection and other STDs	Poor acceptance by some users; latex allergy; not to be used with oil-based lubricants

I. **Diaphragm**
  A. Diaphragms function as a physical barrier and as a reservoir for spermicide. They are particularly acceptable for patients who have only intermittent intercourse. Diaphragms are available in 5-mm incremental sizes from 55 to 80 mm. They must remain in place for eight hours after intercourse and may be damaged by oil-based lubricants.
  B. **Method for fitting a diaphragm**
    1. Selecting a diaphragm may begin by inserting a 70-mm diaphragm (the average size) and then determining whether this size is correct or is too large or too small.
    2. Another method is to estimate the appropriate size by placing a gloved hand in the vagina and using the index and middle fingers to measure the distance from the introitus to the cervix.
II. **Oral contraceptives**
  A. Oral contraceptives have a failure rate of only 3 percent. OCPs have been associated with decreased risks of endometrial and ovarian cancers, benign breast disease, ectopic pregnancy and dysmenorrhea.

Hormonal Content of Selected Oral Contraceptives

Oral contraceptive	Estrogen and progestin content	Constant estrogen dose	Constant progestin dose	Generation
Monophasic agents				
Alesse (available as Alesse-21 or Alesse-28)	20 mcg ethinyl estradiol, 0.1 mg levonorgestrel	Yes	Yes	Second
Loestrin (available as Loestrin 21 1/20 or Loestrin Fe 1/20)	20 mcg ethinyl estradiol, 1.0 mg norethindrone acetate	Yes	Yes	First
Desogen	30 mcg ethinyl estradiol, 0.15 mg desogestrel	Yes	Yes	Third
Levlen	30 mcg ethinyl estradiol, 0.15 mg levonorgestrel	Yes	Yes	Second
Lo/Ovral	30 mcg ethinyl estradiol, 0.3 mg norgestrel	Yes	Yes	First
Nordette	30 mcg ethinyl estradiol, 0.15 mg levonorgestrel	Yes	Yes	Second
Ortho-Cept	30 mcg ethinyl estradiol, 0.15 mg desogestrel	Yes	Yes	Third
Brevicon	35 mcg ethinyl estradiol, 0.5 mg norethindrone	Yes	Yes	First
Demulen 1/35	35 mcg ethinyl estradiol, 1.0 mg ethynodiol diacetate	Yes	Yes	First
Modicon	35 mcg ethinyl estradiol, 0.5 mg norethindrone	Yes	Yes	First
Norethin 1/35E	35 mcg ethinyl estradiol, 1.0 mg norethindrone	Yes	Yes	First
Norinyl 1+35	35 mcg ethinyl estradiol, 1.0 mg norethindrone	Yes	Yes	First
Ortho-Cyclen	35 mcg ethinyl estradiol, 0.25 mg norgestimate	Yes	Yes	Second
Ortho-Novum 1/35	35 mcg ethinyl estradiol, 1.0 mg norethindrone	Yes	Yes	First
Ovcon-35	35 mcg ethinyl estradiol, 0.4 mg norethindrone	Yes	Yes	First
Demulen 1/50	50 mcg ethinyl estradiol, 1.0 mg ethynodiol diacetate	Yes	Yes	First

Oral contra-ceptive	Estrogen and progestin content	Constant estrogen dose	Con-stant proges-tin dose	Genera-tion
Ovcon-50	50 mcg ethinyl estradiol, 1.0 mg norethindrone	Yes	Yes	First
Ovral	50 mcg ethinyl estradiol, 0.5 mg norgestrel	Yes	Yes	First
Norinyl 1+50	50 mcg mestranol, 1.0 mg norethindrone	Yes	Yes	First
Ortho-Novum 1/50	50 mcg mestranol, 1.0 mg norethindrone	Yes	Yes	First
Triphasic agents				
Ortho-Novum 7/7/7	35 mcg ethinyl estradiol, 0.5/0.75/1.0 mg norethindrone	Yes	No	First
Ortho Tri-Cyclen	35 mcg ethinyl estradiol, 0.18/0.215/0.25 mg norgestimate	Yes	No	Second
Tri-Norinyl	35 mcg ethinyl estradiol, 0.5/1.0/0.5 mg norethindrone	Yes	No	First
Tri-Levlen	30/40/30 mcg ethinyl estradiol, 0.05/0.075/0.125 mg levonorgestrel	No	No	Second
Triphasil	30/40/30 mcg ethinyl estradiol, 0.05/0.075/0.125 mg levonorgestrel	No	No	Second
Estrogen phasic agent				
Estrostep (Estrostep 21 or Estrostep Fe)	20/30/35 mcg ethinyl estradiol, 1 mg norethindrone	No	Yes	First
Progestin-only agents				
Micronor	0.35 mg norethindrone	None	Yes	Not ap-plicable
Nor-QD	0.35 mg norethindrone	None	Yes	Not ap-plicable
Ovrette	0.075 mg norgestrel	None	Yes	Not ap-plicable

B. Combination oral contraceptives
   1. Estrogen-progestin oral contraceptives act by inhibiting ovulation through suppression of gonadotropin secretion. Triphasic oral contraceptives decrease the incidence of progestin-related side effects and breakthrough bleeding.

2. Second-generation oral contraceptives contain norgestimate or levonorgestrel as the progestin. Third-generation agents contain desogestrel or gestodene as the progestin. Estrostep is a lower-dose estrogen preparation with varying amounts of estrogen.

Contraindications to Use of Hormonal Contraceptive Methods

Method	Contraindications
Oral combination contraceptive	Active liver disease, hepatic adenoma, thrombophlebitis, history of or active thromboembolic disorder, cardiovascular or cerebrovascular disease, known or suspected breast cancer, undiagnosed abnormal vaginal bleeding, jaundice with past pregnancy or hormone use, pregnancy, breast-feeding, smoking in women over age 35
Progestin-only pill	Undiagnosed abnormal vaginal bleeding, known or suspected breast cancer, cholestatic jaundice of pregnancy or jaundice with previous pill use, hepatic adenoma, known or suspected pregnancy
Depot-medroxyprogesterone acetate (Depo-Provera) injection	Acute liver disease or tumor, thrombophlebitis, known or suspected breast cancer, undiagnosed abnormal vaginal bleeding
Levonorgestrel implant (Norplant)	Acute liver disease or tumor, active thrombophlebitis, known or suspected breast cancer, history of idiopathic intracranial hypertension, undiagnosed abnormal vaginal bleeding, pregnancy, hypersensitivity to any component of the implant system

Side Effects of Hormones Used in Contraceptive Agents

Type of effect	Symptoms
Estrogenic	Nausea, breast tenderness, fluid retention
Progestational	Acne, increased appetite, weight gain, depression, fatigue
Androgenic	Weight gain. hirsutism, acne, oily skin, breakthrough bleeding

3. **Androgenic effects** attributable to progestin include hair growth, male-pattern baldness, nausea, and acne. If such side effects develop, a switch to a second- or third-generation agent with lower androgenic potential may resolve these problems. Women who experience nausea may benefit from taking the medication at night.
4. **Hypertension**, usually less than 5 mm Hg, may occur in some patients. If significant hypertension develops, a lower dose of progestin may be tried.
5. **Weight gain** may be countered by switching to a different formulation.
C. **Administration issues**
   1. If started during the first five days of the menstrual cycle, oral contraceptives are effective throughout the first cycle of use. The medication should be taken at the same time each day.
   2. **Amenorrhea** may occur with long-term use. Administration of an agent

with higher estrogen or lower progestin activity may resolve this problem. A missed menstrual period indicates a need for a pregnancy test.

3. **Breakthrough bleeding** often occurs during the first three months of use. If breakthrough bleeding is a problem, a higher-dose progestin or estrogen agent may be tried. Agents that contain norgestrel are associated with low rates of breakthrough bleeding.

4. **If a woman misses an oral contraceptive dose**, she should take the dose as soon as she remembers it or take two doses the next day and then continue administration of the remainder of the monthly pack as usual. If two doses are missed during the first two weeks of the cycle, two doses per day should be taken for two days, and an additional form of contraception should be used for one week. The remainder of the pack should be administered as usual. If two or more doses are missed during the third week, the pack should be discarded, a new pack should be started, and an additional contraceptive method should be used for one week.

D. Progestin-only agents

1. Progestin-only agents are slightly less effective than combination oral contraceptives. They have failure rates of 0.5 percent compared with the 0.1 percent rate with combination oral contraceptives.

2. Progestin-only oral contraceptives (Micronor, Nor-QD, Ovrette) provide a useful alternative in women who cannot take estrogen and those over age 40. Progestin-only contraception is recommended for nursing mothers. Milk production is unaffected by use of progestin-only agents.

3. If the usual time of ingestion is delayed for more than three hours, an alternative form of birth control should be used for the following 48 hours. Because progestin-only agents are taken continuously, without hormone-free periods, menses may be irregular, infrequent or absent.

III. Medroxyprogesterone acetate injections

A. Depot medroxyprogesterone acetate (Depo-Provera) is an injectable progestin. A 150-mg dose provides 12 weeks of contraception. However, an effective level of contraception is maintained for 14 weeks after an injection. After discontinuation of the injections, resumption of ovulation requires nine months.

B. Every 12 weeks, the medication is given IM. An injection should be administered within five days after the onset of menses or after proof of a negative pregnancy test. Medroxyprogesterone may be administered immediately after childbirth.

C. Medroxyprogesterone injections are a good choice for patients, such as adolescents, who have difficulty remembering to take their oral contraceptive or who have a tendency to use other methods inconsistently. Medroxyprogesterone may also be a useful choice for women who have contraindications to estrogen. This method should not be used for women who desire a rapid return to fertility after discontinuing contraception.

D. Contraindications and side effects

1. Breakthrough bleeding is common during the first few months of use. Most women experience regular bleeding or amenorrhea within six months after the first injection. If breakthrough bleeding persists beyond this period, nonsteroidal anti-inflammatory agents, combination oral contraceptives or a 10- to 21-day course of oral estrogen may eliminate the problem. About 50% of women who have received the injections for one year experience amenorrhea.

2. Side effects include weight gain, headache and dizziness.

IV. Levonorgestrel contraceptive implant (Norplant) is effective for 5 years and consists of six flexible Silastic capsules. Adequate serum levels are obtained within 24 hours after implantation.

V. Emergency contraception

A. Emergency contraception may be considered for a patient who reports a contraceptive failure, such as condom breakage, or other circumstances of unprotected sexual intercourse, such as a sexual assault. If menstruation does not occur within 21 days, a pregnancy test should be performed.

B. Emergency contraception is effective for up to 72 hours after intercourse.

Oral Contraceptives Used for Emergency Contraception

The first two pills should be taken within 72 hours after sexual intercourse, followed 12 hours later by the remaining two pills.

Contraceptive	Pills per dose
Ovral	Two white pills
Alesse (2 or 28-day formulation)	Five pink pills
Levlen	Four light-orange pills
Lo/Ovral	Four white pills
Nordette	Four light-orange pills
Triphasil	Four light-yellow pills
Tri-Levlen	Four light-yellow pills
Preven	Two blue pills

C. The major side effect of emergency contraception with oral contraceptives is nausea, which occurs in 50% of women; vomiting occurs in 20%. If the patient vomits within two hours after ingesting a dose, the dose should be repeated. An antiemetic, such as phenothiazine (Compazine), 5-10 mg PO, or trimethobenzamide (Tigan), 100-250 mg, may be taken one hour before administration of the contraceptive.

VI. Intrauterine devices

A. IUDs represent the most commonly used method of reversible contraception worldwide. The **Progestasert** IUD releases progesterone and must be replaced every 12 months. The **Copper-T** IUD is a copper-containing device which may be used for 10 years.

B. IUDs act by causing a localized foreign-body inflammatory reaction that inhibits implantation of the ovum. An IUD may be a good choice for parous women who are in a monogamous relationship and do not have dysmenorrhea.

C. Contraindications include omen who are at high risk for STDs and those who have a history of pelvic inflammatory disease, and women at high risk for endocarditis. Oral administration of doxycycline, 200 mg, or azithromycin (Zithromax), 500 mg, one hour before insertion reduces the incidence of insertion-related infections.

References: See page 195.

Endometriosis

Ten percent of women will develop endometriosis, characterized by the presence of endometrial tissue at sites outside the uterine cavity, resulting in cyclical dysmenorrhea. The most common sites are the ovaries, posterior cul-de-sac, uterosacral ligaments, posterior broad ligament, and anterior cul-de-sac. The uterine serosa, rectovaginal septum, cervix, vagina, rectosigmoid, and bladder are less frequent locations.

I. **Clinical manifestations**
   A. Endometriosis is characterized by cyclical pain, usually beginning prior to menses. Deep dyspareunia and sacral backache with menses are common.
   B. Infertility is a frequent consequence of endometriosis. Premenstrual tenesmus or diarrhea may indicate rectosigmoid endometriosis. Cyclic dysuria or hematuria may indicate bladder endometriosis.
   C. Tender nodules are often palpable through the posterior vaginal fornix on bimanual examination and along the uterosacral ligaments on rectovaginal examination. Ovarian enlargement, fixation of the adnexal structures, and uterine retrodisplacement may also be detected.
   D. Ultrasound may identify adnexal masses. Endometriosis can be definitively diagnosed only by laparoscopy.

II. **Treatment of endometriosis**
   A. Initial therapy consists of a nonsteroidal anti-inflammatory drug.
      1. Naproxen (Naprosyn) 500 mg followed by 250 mg PO tid-qid prn [250, 375,500 mg].
      2. Naproxen sodium (Aleve) 200 mg PO tid prn.
      3. Naproxen sodium (Anaprox) 550 mg, followed by 275 mg PO tid-qid prn.
      4. Ibuprofen (Motrin) 800 mg, then 400 mg PO q4-6h prn.
      5. Mefenamic acid (Ponstel) 500 mg PO followed by 250 mg q6h prn.
   B. **Combined estrogen-progestin.** Low-dose, combination, monophasic birth control pills often relieve mild to moderate pelvic pain; they are often taken continuously.
   C. **Progestin-only regimen.** Medroxyprogesterone (Provera), 10-30 mg/d, produces significant pain relief; breakthrough bleeding is common. Depo-Provera may be used unless fertility is desired in the near future.
   D. **Gonadotropin-releasing hormone agonists**
      1. GnRH agonists inhibit gonadal function, resulting in hypoestrogenism. Pain is relieved in most patients by the second or third month.
      2. Intramuscular leuprolide 3.75 mg once monthly or nafarelin, 200 mg nasal spray twice daily for 3-6 months may be used.
      3. Side effects, such as osteoporosis, hot flashes, headaches, and depression, are common. Symptoms recur after discontinuation of therapy in most patients.
   E. **Surgical therapy.** Endometriosis is usually treated surgically at the time of diagnosis by laparoscopic cautery. Hysterectomy with bilateral oophorectomy is the definitive treatment for endometriosis.

References: See page 195.

Premenstrual Syndrome

Premenstrual syndrome (PMS) affects 5-10% of reproductive-age women. Ovarian steroids play an important role in symptomogenesis, since studies have shown that oophorectomy and gonadotropin-releasing hormone (GnRH) agonists resolve symptoms. Whole blood serotonin (5-HT) has been shown to be low during the luteal phase in patients with PMS.

Symptoms of Premenstrual Syndrome

Mood
  Depression
  Hostility
  Irritability
  Mood swings
  Negative world view
  Sadness
Behavioral
  Arguing
  Decreased interest in anything
  Hyperphagia

Somatic
  Appetite changes
  Bloating
  Carbohydrate craving
  Fatigue
  Headache
  Hot flashes
  Insomnia
  Mastalgia
Cognitive
  Confusion
  Poor concentration

DSM-IV Criteria for Premenstrual Dysphoric Disorder

- Five or more symptoms
- At least one of the following four symptoms:
    Markedly depressed mood, feelings of hopelessness, or self-depre-
    cating thoughts
    Marked anxiety, tension, feeling of being "keyed up" or "on edge"
    Marked affective lability
    Persistent and marked anger or irritability or increase in interpersonal
    conflicts
- Additional symptoms that may be used to fulfill the criteria:
    Decreased interest in usual activities
    Subjective sense of difficulty in concentrating
    Lethargy, easy fatigability, or marked lack of energy
    Marked change in appetite, overeating, or specific food cravings
    Hypersomnia or insomnia
    Subjective sense of being overwhelmed or out of control
- Other physical symptoms such as breast tenderness or swelling,
  headaches, joint or muscle pain, a sensation of bloating, or weight gain
- Symptoms occurring during last week of luteal phase
- Symptoms are absent postmenstrually
- Disturbances that interfere with work or school or with usual social
  activities and relationships
- Disturbances that are not an exacerbation of symptoms of another
  disorder

I. Clinical evaluation of PMS

A. PMS involves an assortment of disabling physical and emotional symptoms
   that appear during the luteal phase and resolve within the first week of the
   follicular phase. Symptoms of PMS fall into four main categories: mood,
   somatic, cognitive, and behavioral.

B. No specific serum marker can be used to confirm the diagnosis.
   Premenstrual dysphoric disorder is diagnosed when mood symptoms
   predominate symptoms of PMS.

C. The differential diagnosis includes hypothyroidism, anemia, perimenopause,
   drug and alcohol abuse, and affective disorders. Common alternative
   diagnoses in patients complaining of PMS include affective or personality
   disorder, menopausal symptoms, eating disorder, and alcohol or other
   substance abuse. A medical condition such as diabetes or hypothyroidism,
   is the cause of the symptoms in 8.4%, and 10.6% have symptoms related

to oral contraceptive (OC) use.

II. Treatment of premenstrual syndrome

A. More than 70% of women with PMS will respond to therapy.

B. Symptomatic treatment

1. **Fluid retention and bloating** may be relieved by limiting salty foods. If 5 pounds or more are gained during the luteal phase, diuretic therapy may be effective. Spironolactone (Aldactone) is the drug of choice because of its potassium-sparing effects. The dose ranges from 25-200 mg qd during the luteal phase.

2. **Mastalgia.** Support bras, decreased caffeine intake, nutritional supplements (evening primrose oil or vitamin E, 400 IU), a low-fat diet, oral contraceptives, or non-steroidal anti-inflammatory drugs (NSAIDs) are effective. Bromocriptine (Parlodel), 1.25-2.5 mg po each day of the luteal phase may be effective. Side effects include dizziness and gastrointestinal upset. Other therapies include danazol (Danocrine) 200 mg qd, and tamoxifen (Nolvadex), 10 mg qd for 3 months.

3. **Sleep disturbances**. Conservative measures include regulating sleep patterns, avoiding stimulating events before bedtime, and progressive relaxation and biofeedback therapy. Doxepin (Sinequan), 10-25 mg hs, also is effective.

Treatment for Premenstrual Syndrome

Serotonin-mediated
Fluoxetine (Prozac) 5-20 mg qd
Sertraline (Zoloft) 25-50 mg qd
Paroxetine (Paxil) 5-20 mg qd
Fluvoxamine (LuVox) 25-50 mg qd
Clomipramine (Anafranil) 25-100 mg qhs
Buspirone (BuSpar) 25 mg qd in divided doses

GABA-mediated
Alprazolam (Xanax) 0.25-0.50 mg tid

Mefenamic acid (Ponstel) 250 mg tid with meals
Ovarian suppression
  Ovulation suppression
    Medroxyprogesterone (Provera) 30 mg PO qd
    Medroxyprogesterone acetate injection (Depot-Provera) 150 mg IM q 3 months
    Oral contraceptives
  Total suppression
    Leuprolide (Lupron) 3.75 mg IM each month
    Nafarelin (Synarel) 400-800 pq intranasally qd
    Danazol (Danocrine) 200 mg qd-bid
    Oophorectomy

Vitamin and mineral supplements
Calcium, 600 mg bid, may help decrease negative mood, fluid retention, and pain
Evening primrose oil, 500 mg tid
Magnesium may help decrease negative mood, fluid retention, and pain
Vitamin E, 400 IU qd

Other
    Bromocriptine (Parlodel), 1.25-2.5 mg po each day of the luteal phase
    for breast pain
    Spirolactone (Aldactone) 25-200 mg qd
    Tamoxifen citrate (Nolvadex),10 mg qd for 3 months for breast pain

    4. **Menstrual migraines** often occur just before and during menses.
    Menstrual migraines are treated with NSAIDs. Sumatriptan (Imitrex), 50
    mg po or 30-60 mg intramuscularly (IM); propranolol (Inderal), 80-240
    mg in divided doses; or amitriptyline (Elavil), 25-100 mg, taken before
    bedtime.
III. Syndromal treatment
  A. Nonpharmacologic remedies include calcium (600 mg bid) and magnesium
    (360 mg qd), possibly with the addition of vitamins.
  B. SSRIs are appropriate for women with mood symptoms. Cyclical luteal
    phase administration of fluoxetine (Prozac), 20 mg, or sertraline (Zoloft),
    25-50 mg, has shown efficacy. Initially, SSRIs should be restricted to the
    luteal phase of each cycle. If the patient's symptoms are not ameliorated
    after a trial of 2-3 months, SSRIs can be given throughout the cycle.

Lifestyle Modifications That Help Relieve Premenstrual Syndrome

Moderate, regular, aerobic exercise (1-2 miles of brisk walking 4-5
times/week) may decrease depression and pain symptoms

Reducing or eliminating salt and alcohol, especially in the luteal phase;
eating small, frequent meas; increasing complex carbohydrates

  C. Anxiolytics and antidepressants. Alprazolam (Xanax), 0.25-0.5 mg tid,
    given during the luteal phase only may relieve anxiety. Dependence is
    possible, but restricting the agent to the luteal period may help a subset of
    women.
  D. Ovulation suppression
    1. Less complex hormonal therapies include OCs and progestins. OCs
    (especially triphasic formulations) may decrease the cyclical symptoms
    of PMS, although they may worsen symptoms in a subset of patients.
    2. **Medroxyprogesterone acetate (Provera),** 30 mg PO qd, may alleviate
    symptoms. Once the symptoms resolve, drug therapy may be switched
    to medroxyprogesterone acetate injections (Depot-Provera), 150 mg IM,
    every 3 months.
    3. Ovarian suppression with GnRH agonists induces menopause. PMS
    symptoms will be relieved, but patients experience menopausal side
    effects, including irritability, insomnia, hot flashes, and vaginal dryness.
    To prevent osteoporosis, add-back therapy with estrogen and proges-
    terone is required.
    4. **Leuprolide (Lupron Depot),** 3.75 mg IM each month, or nafarelin
    (Synarel), 400-800 pg qd intranasally are effective. Conjugated equine
    estrogen, 0.625 mg, with medroxyprogesterone acetate, 2.5 mg given
    daily will provide adequate estrogen for cardioprotection and shield the
    bones from calcium breakdown.
    5. **Danazol,** 200 mg qd-bid, is effective in decreasing the symptoms of
    PMS. Side effects include hirsutism, acne, and weight gain.
    6. **Surgery.** Oophorectomy is reserved for patients whose symptoms have
    resolved completely for 4-6 months with GnRH agonists, who have
    completed child bearing, and who require more than 5 years of long-term

suppression.

References: See page 195.

Amenorrhea

Amenorrhea may be associated with infertility, endometrial hyperplasia, or osteopenia. It may be the presenting sign of an underlying metabolic, endocrine, congenital, or gynecologic disorder.

I. **Pathophysiology of amenorrhea**
   A. Amenorrhea may be caused by failure of the hypothalamic-pituitary-gonadal axis, by absence of end organs, or by obstruction of the outflow tract.
   B. **Menses** usually occur at intervals of 28 (±3) days, with a normal range of 18-40 days.
   C. **Amenorrhea** is defined as the absence of menstruation for 3 or more months in a women with past menses (secondary amenorrhea) or the absence of menarche by age 16 in girls who have never menstruated (primary amenorrhea). Pregnancy is the most common cause of amenorrhea.

II. **Clinical evaluation of amenorrhea**
   A. **Menstrual history** should include the age of menarche, last menstrual period, and previous menstrual pattern. Diet, medications, and psychologic stress should be assessed.
   B. **Galactorrhea**, previous radiation therapy, chemotherapy, or recent weight gain or loss may provide important clues.
   C. **Prolonged, intense exercise**, often associated with dieting, can lead to amenorrhea. Symptoms of decreased estrogen include hot flushes and night sweats.
   D. **Physical examination**
      1. **Breast development and pubic hair distribution** should be assessed because they demonstrate exposure to estrogens and sexual maturity. Galactorrhea is a sign of hyperprolactinemia.
      2. **Thyroid gland** should be palpated for enlargement and nodules. Abdominal striae in a nulliparous woman suggests hypercortisolism (Cushing's syndrome).
      3. **Hair distribution** may reveal signs of androgen excess. The absence of both axillary and pubic hair in a phenotypically normal female suggests androgen insensitivity.
      4. **External genitalia and vagina** should be inspected for atrophy from estrogen deficiency or clitoromegaly from androgen excess. An imperforate hymen or vaginal septum can block the outflow tract.
      5. **Palpation of the uterus and ovaries** assures their presence and detects abnormalities.

III. **Diagnostic approach to amenorrhea**
   A. Menstrual flow requires an intact hypothalamic-pituitary-ovarian axis, a hormonally responsive uterus, and an intact outflow tract. The evaluation should localize the abnormality to either the uterus, ovary, anterior pituitary, or hypothalamus.
   B. **Step one--exclude pregnancy.** Pregnancy is the most common cause of secondary amenorrhea, and it must be excluded with a pregnancy test.
   C. **Step two--exclude hyperthyroidism and hyperprolactinemia**
      1. **Hypothyroidism and hyperprolactinemia** can cause amenorrhea. These disorders are excluded with a serum thyroid-stimulating hormone (TSH) and prolactin.
      2. **Hyperprolactinemia.** Prolactin inhibits the secretion of gonadotropin-releasing hormone. One-third of women with no obvious cause of amenorrhea have hyperprolactinemia. Mildly elevated prolactin levels

should be confirmed by repeat testing and review the patient's medications. Hyperprolactinemia requires an MRI to exclude a pituitary tumor.

Drugs Associated with Amenorrhea	
Drugs that Increase Prolactin	Antipsychotics Tricyclic antidepressants Calcium channel blockers
Drugs with Estrogenic Activity	Digoxin, marijuana, oral contraceptives
Drugs with Ovarian Toxicity	Chemotherapeutic agents

D. Step three--assess estrogen status
   1. **The progesterone challenge test** is used to determine estrogen status and determine the competence of the uterine outflow tract.
   2. Medroxyprogesterone (Provera) 10 mg is given PO qd for 10 consecutive days. Uterine bleeding within 2-7 days after completion is considered a positive test. A positive result suggests chronic anovulation, rather than hypothalamic-pituitary insufficiency or ovarian failure, and a positive test also confirms the presence of a competent outflow tract.
   3. A negative test indicates either an incompetent outflow tract, nonreactive endometrium, or inadequate estrogen stimulation.
      a. To rule out an abnormality of the outflow tract, a regimen of conjugated estrogens (Premarin), 1.25 mg daily on days 1 through 21 of the cycle, is prescribed. Medroxyprogesterone (Provera) 10 mg is given on the last 5 days of the 21-day cycle. (A combination oral contraceptive agent can also be used.)
      b. Withdrawal bleeding within 2-7 days of the last dose of progesterone confirms the presence of an unobstructed outflow tract and a normal endometrium, and the problem is localized to the hypothalamic-pituitary axis or ovaries.
   4. In patients who have had prolonged amenorrhea, an endometrial biopsy should be considered before withdrawal bleeding is induced. Biopsy can reveal endometrial hyperplasia.
E. Step four--evaluation of hypoestrogenic amenorrhea
   1. Serum follicle-stimulating hormone (FSH) and luteinizing hormone (LH) levels should be measured to localize the problem to the ovary, pituitary or hypothalamus.
   2. Ovarian failure
      a. An FSH level greater than 50 mIU/mL indicates ovarian failure.
      b. Ovarian failure is considered "premature" when it occurs in women less than 40 years of age.
   3. Pituitary or hypothalamic dysfunction
      a. A normal or low gonadotropin level is indicative of pituitary or hypothalamic failure. An MRI is the most sensitive study to rule out a pituitary tumor.
      b. If MRI does not reveal a tumor, a defect in pulsatile GnRH release from the hypothalamus is the probable cause.
IV. Management of chronic anovulation
   A. Adequate estrogen and anovulation is indicated by withdrawal bleeding with the progesterone challenge test.
   B. Often there is a history of weight loss, psychosocial stress, or excessive exercise. Women usually have a normal or low body weight and normal secondary sex characteristics.

1. Reducing stress and assuring adequate nutrition may induce ovulation.
2. These women are at increased risk for endometrial cancer because of the hyperplastic effect of unopposed estrogen.
3. Progesterone (10 mg/day for the first 7-10 days of every month) is given to induce withdrawal bleeding. If contraception is desired, a low-dose oral contraceptive should be used.

V. Management of hypothalamic dysfunction

A. Amenorrheic women with a normal prolactin level, a negative progesterone challenge, with low or normal gonadotropin levels, and with a normal sella turcica imaging are considered to have hypothalamic dysfunction.

B. Hypothalamic amenorrhea usually results from psychologic stress, depression, severe weight loss, anorexia nervosa, or strenuous exercise.

C. Hypoestrogenic women are at risk for osteoporosis and cardiovascular disease. Oral contraceptives are appropriate in young women. Women not desiring contraception should take estrogen, 0.625 mg, with medroxyprogesterone (Provera) 2.5 mg, every day of the month. Calcium and vitamin D supplementation are also recommended.

VI. Management of disorders of the outflow tract or uterus--intrauterine adhesions (Asherman syndrome)

A. Asherman syndrome is the most common outflow-tract abnormality that causes amenorrhea. This disorder should be considered if amenorrhea develops following curettage or after endometritis.

B. Hysterosalpingography will detect adhesions. Therapy consists of hysteroscopy and lysis of adhesions.

VII. Management of disorders of the ovaries

A. Ovarian failure is suspected if menopausal symptoms are present. Women with premature ovarian failure who are less than 30 years of age should undergo karyotyping to rule out the presence of a Y chromosome. If a Y chromosome is detected, testicular tissue should be removed.

B. Patients with ovarian failure should be prescribed estrogen 0.625 mg with progesterone 2.5 mg daily with calcium and vitamin D.

VIII. Disorders of the anterior pituitary

A. Prolactin-secreting adenoma are excluded by MRI of the pituitary.

B. Cabergoline (Dostinex) or bromocriptine (Parlodel) are used for most adenomas; surgery is considered later.

References: See page 195.

Breast Disorders

I. Nipple Discharge

A. Clinical evaluation

1. Nipple discharge may be a sign of cancer, and it must be thoroughly evaluated. Eight percent of biopsies performed for nipple discharge demonstrate cancer.

2. Determine the duration, bilaterality or unilaterality of the discharge, and the presence of blood. A history of oral contraceptives, hormone preparations, phenothiazines, nipple or breast stimulation, or lactation should be determined. Discharges that flow spontaneously are more likely to be pathologic than discharges that must be manually expressed.

3. Unilateral, pink colored, bloody or non-milky discharge, or discharges associated with a mass are the discharges of most concern.

4. Bilateral, milky discharge suggest an endocrine problem. Nipple discharge secondary to malignancy is more likely to occur in older patients.

5. **Risk factors.** A risk assessment should identify risk factors, including age over 50 years, past personal history of breast cancer, history of

hyperplasia on previous breast biopsies, and family history of breast cancer in a first-degree relative (mother, sister, daughter).

B. Physical examination should include inspection of the breast for ulceration or contour changes and inspection of the nipple. Palpation should be performed with the patient in both the upright and the supine positions to determine the presence of a mass.

C. Diagnostic evaluation
1. **Bloody discharge.** A mammogram of the involved breast should be obtained if the patient is over 35 years old and has not had a mammogram within the preceding 6 months. Biopsy of any suspicious lesions should be completed.
2. **Watery, unilateral discharge** should be referred to a surgeon for evaluation and possible biopsy.
3. **Non-bloody discharge** should be tested for the presence of blood with standard Hemoccult cards. Nipple discharge secondary to carcinoma usually contains hemoglobin.
4. **Milky bilateral discharge** should be evaluated with assays of prolactin and thyroid stimulating hormone to exclude an endocrinologic cause.
   a. A mammogram should also be performed if the patient is due for routine mammographic screening.
   b. If results of the mammogram and the endocrinologic screening studies are normal, the patient should return for a follow-up visit in 6 months to ensure that there has been no specific change in the character of the discharge, such as development of bleeding.

II. Breast Pain
A. Determine the duration and location of the pain, associated trauma, previous breast surgery, associated lumps, or nipple discharge.

B. Pain is an uncommon presenting symptom for breast cancer; however, cancer must be excluded. Cancer is the etiology in 5% of patients with breast pain. Pain that is associated with breast cancer is usually unilateral, intense, and constant.

C. Patients less than 35 years of age without a mass
1. It is unlikely that the pain is a symptom of cancer.
2. A follow-up clinical breast examination should be performed in 1-2 months. Diagnostic mammography is usually not helpful but may be considered.

D. Patient 35 years of age or older
1. Obtain diagnostic mammogram, and obtain an ultrasound if a cystic lesion is present.
2. If studies are negative, a follow-up examination in 1-2 months is appropriate. If a suspicious lesion is detected, biopsy is required.

E. Mastodynia
1. Mastodynia is defined as breast pain in the absence of a mass or other pathologic abnormality.
2. **Causes of mastodynia** include menstrually related pain, costochondritis, trauma, and sclerosing adenosis.

III. Fibrocystic Complex
A. Breast changes are usually multifocal, bilateral, and diffuse. One or more isolated fibrocystic lumps or areas of asymmetry may be present. The areas are usually tender.

B. This disorder predominantly occurs in women with premenstrual abnormalities, nulliparous women, and nonusers of oral contraceptives.

C. The disorder usually begins in mid-20's or early 30's. Tenderness is associated with menses and lasts about a week. The upper outer quadrant of the breast is most frequently involved bilaterally. There is no increased risk of cancer for the majority of patients.

D. Suspicious areas may be evaluated by fine needle aspiration (FNA) cytology. If mammography and FNA are negative for cancer, and the clinical

examination is benign, open biopsy is generally not needed.
  E. **Medical management of fibrocystic complex**
     1. **Oral contraceptives** are effective for severe breast pain in most young women. Start with a pill that contains low amounts of estrogen and relatively high amounts of progesterone (Loestrin, LoOvral, Ortho-Cept).
     2. If oral contraceptives do not provide relief, medroxyprogesterone 5-10 mg/day from days 15-25 of each cycle is added.
     3. A professionally fitted support bra often provides significant relief.
     4. A low fat diet, vitamins (E and B complex), evening primrose oil, and stopping smoking may provide relief.
     5. NSAIDs and bromocriptine have been used.

References: See page 195.

Menopause

The average age of menopause is 51 years, with a range of 41-55. Menopause occurs before age 40 in about 5% of women. Ovarian production of estrogen is significantly reduced, leading to hot flushes, mood disturbances, thinning of genitourinary tissues, loss of calcium from the skeleton, a metabolic shift to a more atherogenic lipoprotein profile, and an elevated follicle-stimulating hormone (FSH) level greater than 40 mIU/mL.
I. **Benefits of hormone replacement therapy**
   A. **Central nervous System symptoms**
      1. Changes in neurologic function such as increased irritability, mood disorders, mild depression, hot flushes, and sleep disturbances may arise during the perimenopausal transition. Estrogen replacement therapy is the most effective treatment for hot flushes. Hormone replacement with estrogen may help to reverse cognitive changes and improve function.
      2. In elderly menopausal women, estrogens may retard the progression of dementia, especially Alzheimer's disease.
   B. **Sexual function.** Libido may decrease at the time of the menopause. The use of testosterone with estrogen may induce a positive effect on mood and overall sense of well-being, particularly in women who have had their ovaries removed.
   C. **Cardiovascular symptoms.** Coronary heart disease is the leading cause of death in women. Estrogens protect against coronary heart disease by lowering LDL cholesterol and increasing HDL cholesterol concentrations. Estrogen may also provide arterial vasodilation and increased perfusion.
   D. **Osteoporosis**
      1. Bone loss in women accelerates at the onset of menopause on average at a rate of approximately 3% per year for the first 5 years and 1% per year thereafter. Hip fractures frequently occur 15-25 years after menopause and result from the reduced bone mass. Other fractures associated with osteoporosis include fractures of the vertebrae, distal forearm, and proximal humerus.
      2. Osteoporosis is diagnosed when bone mineral density decreases to less than 2.5 standard deviations below the young adult peak mean. Estrogen therapy has been shown to be effective in preventing bone loss.
   E. **Genitourinary symptoms.** Withdrawal of estradiol during menopause results in thinning of the mucosal layer. The vaginal and urethral mucosa appear pale, dry, and flattened. These changes are associated with vaginal dryness, dyspareunia, atrophic vaginitis, urethritis, and urinary incontinence. Use of systemic estrogen replacement or local estrogen creams and urethral suppositories can reverse these changes.

II. Risk factors associated with hormone replacement therapy

A. **Endometrial hyperplasia and endometrial cancer.** Long-term use of estrogen alone has been associated with the development of endometrial hyperplasia and endometrial cancer. In women with a uterus, progestin therapy protects the endometrium from hyperplastic transformation during estrogen replacement therapy

B. **Breast cancer**
  1. An increased risk of breast cancer has been associated with the extended duration of endogenous estrogen exposure such as that which occurs with early menarche, late menopause, and obesity.
  2. Some evidence suggests a small increase in breast cancer risk after 10-15 years of estrogen supplementation. No consistent link between hormone replacement therapy and breast cancer has been found. Because women with prior breast cancer have an increased risk for a second primary breast cancer, close surveillance is warranted.

III. Therapeutic options

A. **Contraindications to hormone replacement therapy:** Family or individual history of breast cancer; estrogen dependent neoplasia; undiagnosed genital bleeding; and a history of or active thromboembolic disorder.

B. Hormone replacement therapy should be considered to relieve vasomotor symptoms, genital urinary tract atrophy, mood and cognitive disturbances, and to prevent osteoporosis and cardiovascular disease. It also may be considered to help prevent colon cancer, Alzheimer's disease, and adult tooth loss.

C. Effective doses of estrogen for the prevention of osteoporosis are: 0.625 mg of conjugated estrogen, 0.5 mg of micronized estradiol, and 0.3 mg of esterified estrogen.

D. In those women with a uterus, a progestin should be given either continuously (2.5 mg of medroxyprogesterone acetate per day) or in a sequential fashion (5-10 mg of medroxyprogesterone (Provera) for 12-14 days each month).

E. **Combination estrogen with progestin (Prempro),** 0.625 mg of estrogen and 2.5 mg of medroxyprogesterone, one tablet every day.

F. **Estrogen cream.** Application 1/4 of an applicator(0.6 mg) daily for 1-2 weeks, then 2-3 times/week will usually relieve urogenital symptoms. This regimen is used concomitantly with oral estrogen.

G. **Treatment of low libido** consists of micronized testosterone cream (1 mg/mL) applied to the inner surface of both forearms daily. Start with 1 mg/day and increase to 2.5 mg/day if necessary.

References: See page 195.

Osteoporosis

Osteoporosis is a common cause of skeletal fractures, which occur primarily at the wrist, the spine, or the hip. Bone loss accelerates during menopause due to the decrease in estrogen production. Approximately 20% of women have osteoporosis in their seventh decade of life, 30% of women in their eighth decade of life, and 70% of women older than 80 years.

I. Diagnosis

A. **Risk factors** for osteoporosis include female gender, increasing age, family history, Caucasian or Asian race, estrogen deficient state, nulliparity, sedentarism, lifelong history of low calcium intake, smoking, excessive alcohol or caffeine consumption, and use of glucocorticoid drugs. Patients who have already sustained a fragility fracture have a markedly increased risk of sustaining further fractures.

B. **Bone density testing.** Bone density is the strongest predictor of fracture risk. Bone density can be assessed by dual X-ray absorptiometry.

Indications for Bone Density Testing

Estrogen-deficient women at clinical risk for osteoporosis
Individuals with vertebral abnormalities
Individuals receiving, or planning to receive, long-term glucocorticoid
(steroid) therapy
Individuals with primary hyperparathyroidism
Individuals being monitored to assess the response of an approved
osteoporosis drug therapy

II. **Prevention and treatment strategies**
   A. A balanced diet including 1000-1500 mg of calcium, weight bearing exercise, and avoidance of alcohol and tobacco products should be encouraged. Daily calcium supplementation (1000-1500 mg) along with 400-800 IU vitamin D should be recommended.
   B. Females who are not willing or incapable of receiving estrogen therapy and have osteopenic bone densities may consider alternative agents such as alendronate and raloxifene. After the age of 65, a bone density test should be performed to decide if pharmacologic therapy should be considered to prevent or treat osteoporosis.

Drugs for Osteoporosis

Drug	Dosage	Indication	Comments
Estrogen	0.625 mg qd with medroxy-progesterone (Provera), 2.5 mg qd	Prevention and Treatment	
Raloxifene (Evista)	60 mg PO QD	Prevention	No breast or uterine tissue stimulation. Decrease in cholesterol similar to estrogen.
Alendronate (Fosamax)	5 mg PO QD 10 mg PO QD	Prevention Treatment	Take in the morning with 2-3 glasses of water, at least 30 min before any food, beverages, or medication. Reduction in fracture risk.
Calcitonin	200 IU QD (nasal) 50-100 IU QD SQ	Treatment	Modest analgesic effect. Not indicated in the early post-menopausal years.
Calcium	1000-1500 mg/day	Prevention/Treatment	Calcium alone may not prevent osteoporosis
Vitamin D	400-800 IU QD	Prevention/Treatment	May help reduce hip fracture incidence

C. Estrogen replacement therapy
1. All postmenopausal women without contraindications should consider ERT. Contraindications include a family or individual history of breast cancer; estrogen dependent neoplasia; undiagnosed genital bleeding; and a history of or active thromboembolic disorder.
2. ERT should be initiated at the onset of menopause. Conjugated estrogens, at a dose of 0.625 mg per day, result in increases in bone density of 5%.
3. **Bone density assessment** at regular intervals (possibly every 3-5 years) provides density data to help determine if continuation of ERT may be further recommended. If ERT is discontinued and no other therapies are instituted, serial bone density measurements should be continued to monitor bone loss.
4. ERT doubles the risk of endometrial cancer in women with an intact uterus. This increased risk can be eliminated by the addition of medroxyprogesterone (Provera) either cyclically (12-14 days/month) at a dose of 5-10 mg or continuously at a dose of 2.5 mg daily.
5. Other adverse effects related to ERT are breast tenderness, weight gain, headaches, and libido changes. Some evidence suggests a small increase in breast cancer risk after 10-15 years of estrogen supplementation.

D. Selective estrogen receptor modulators
1. Selective estrogen receptor modulators (SERMs) act as estrogen analogs. Tamoxifen is approved for the prevention of breast cancer in patients with a strong family history of breast cancer. Tamoxifen prevents bone loss at the spine.
2. **Raloxifene (Evista)**
   a. **Raloxifene** is approved for the prevention of osteoporosis. When used at 60 mg per day, raloxifene demonstrates modest increases (1.5-2% in 24 months) in bone density. This increase in density is half of that seen in those patients receiving ERT. Raloxifene also results in a beneficial effect on the lipid profile similar to that seen with estrogen.
   b. Raloxifene lacks breast stimulation properties, and it may provide a protective effect against breast cancer, resulting in a 50-70% reduction in breast cancer risk.
   c. Minor common side effects include hot flashes and leg cramps. Serious side effects include an increased risk of venous thromboembolism.

E. Bisphosphonates–alendronate (Fosamax)
1. Alendronate is an oral bisphosphonate approved for the treatment and prevention of osteoporosis. Alendronate exerts its effect on bone by inhibiting osteoclasts.
2. The dose for prevention of osteoporosis is 5 mg per day. This dose results in significant increases in densities of 2-3.5%, similar to those observed in ERT. The dose for treatment of osteoporosis is 10 mg per day. Alendronate provides an approximate 50% reduction in fracture risk at both skeletal sites.
3. Patients should take the pill in the morning with 2-3 glasses of water, at least 30 minutes before any food or beverages. No other medication should be taken at the same time, particularly calcium preparations. Patients should not lie down after taking alendronate to avoid gastroesophageal reflux. Contraindicated include severe renal insufficiency and hypocalcemia.

References: See page 195.

Abnormal Vaginal Bleeding

Menorrhagia (excessive bleeding) is most commonly caused by anovulatory menstrual cycles. Occasionally it is caused by thyroid dysfunction, infections or cancer.

I. Pathophysiology of normal menstruation

A. In response to gonadotropin-releasing hormone from the hypothalamus, the pituitary gland synthesizes follicle-stimulating hormone (FSH) and luteinizing hormone (LH), which induce the ovaries to produce estrogen and progesterone.

B. During the follicular phase, estrogen stimulation causes an increase in endometrial thickness. After ovulation, progesterone causes endometrial maturation. Menstruation is caused by estrogen and progesterone withdrawal.

C. **Abnormal bleeding** is defined as bleeding that occurs at intervals of less than 21 days, more than 36 days, lasting longer than 7 days, or blood loss greater than 80 mL.

II. Clinical evaluation of abnormal vaginal bleeding

A. A menstrual and reproductive history is obtained, including last menstrual period, regularity, duration, frequency; the number of pads used per day, and intermenstrual bleeding.

B. Stress, exercise, weight changes and systemic diseases, particularly thyroid, renal or hepatic diseases, or coagulopathies should be sought. The method of birth control should be determined.

C. Pregnancy complications, such as spontaneous abortion, ectopic pregnancy, placenta previa and abruptio placentae, can cause heavy bleeding. Pregnancy should always be considered as a possible cause of abnormal vaginal bleeding.

III. Puberty and adolescence--menarche to age 16

A. Irregularity is normal during the first few months of menstruation; however, soaking more than 25 pads or 30 tampons during a menstrual period is abnormal.

B. Absence of premenstrual symptoms (breast tenderness, bloating, cramping) is associated with anovulatory cycles.

C. Fever, particularly in association with pelvic or abdominal pain may, indicate pelvic inflammatory disease. A history of easy bruising suggests a coagulation defect. Headaches and visual changes suggest a pituitary tumor.

D. **Physical findings**

1. Pallor not associated with tachycardia or signs of hypovolemia suggests chronic excessive blood loss secondary to anovulatory bleeding, adenomyosis, uterine myomas, or blood dyscrasia.

2. Signs of impending shock indicate that the blood loss is related to pregnancy (including ectopic), trauma, sepsis, or neoplasia.

3. Pelvic masses may represent pregnancy, uterine or ovarian neoplasia, or a pelvic abscess or hematoma.

4. Fever, leukocytosis, and pelvic tenderness suggests PID.

5. Fine, thinning hair, and hypoactive reflexes suggest hypothyroidism.

6. Ecchymoses or multiple bruises may indicate trauma, coagulation defects, medication use, or dietary extremes.

E. **Laboratory tests**

1. CBC and platelet count and a urine or serum pregnancy test should be obtained.

2. Screening for sexually transmitted diseases, thyroid function, and coagulation disorders (partial thromboplastin time, INR, bleeding time) is necessary.

3. **Endometrial sampling** is rarely necessary for those under age 20.

F   Treatment of infrequent bleeding
1. Therapy should be directed at the underlying cause when possible.
2. If the CBC and other initial laboratory tests are normal and the history and physical examination are normal, reassurance is usually all that is necessary.
3. Ferrous gluconate, 325 mg bid-tid, should be prescribed.

G. Treatment of frequent or heavy bleeding
1. Treatment with nonsteroidal anti-inflammatory drugs (NSAIDs) improves platelet aggregation and increases uterine vasoconstriction. NSAIDs are the first choice in the treatment of menorrhagia because they are well tolerated and do not have the hormonal effects of oral contraceptives.
   a. Mefenamic acid (Ponstel) 500 mg tid during the menstrual period.
   b. Naproxen (Anaprox, Naprosyn) 500-mg loading dose, then 250 mg tid during the menstrual period.
   c. Ibuprofen (Motrin, Nuprin) 400-600 mg tid during the menstrual period.
   d. Gastrointestinal distress is common, and NSAIDs are contraindicated in renal failure and peptic ulcer disease.
2. Iron should also be added as ferrous gluconate 325 mg tid.

H. Patients with hypovolemia or a hemoglobin level below 7 g/dL should be hospitalized for hormonal therapy, iron replacement, and possibly transfusion.
1. Hormonal therapy consists of estrogen (Premarin) 25 mg IV q6h until bleeding stops. Thereafter, oral contraceptive pills should be administered q6h x 7 days, then taper slowly to one pill qd.
2. If bleeding continues, IV vasopressin (DDAVP) should be administered. Hysteroscopy may be necessary, and dilation and curettage is a last resort.
3. Iron should also be added as ferrous gluconate 325 mg tid.

IV. Primary childbearing years--ages 16 to early 40's
A. Contraceptive complications and pregnancy are the most common causes of abnormal bleeding in this age group. Anovulation accounts for 20% of cases.
B. Adenomyosis, endometriosis, and fibroids increase in frequency as a woman ages, as do endometrial hyperplasia and endometrial polyps. Pelvic inflammatory disease and endocrine dysfunction may also occur.
C. Laboratory tests
1. CBC and platelet count, Pap smear, and pregnancy test.
2. Screening for sexually transmitted diseases, thyroid dysfunction, and coagulation disorders (partial thromboplastin time, INR, bleeding time).
3. If a non-pregnant woman has a pelvic mass, evaluation is required with ultrasonography or hysterosonography (with uterine saline infusion).
D. Endometrial sampling
1. Long-term unopposed estrogen stimulation in anovulatory patients can result in endometrial hyperplasia, which can progress to adenocarcinoma; therefore, in perimenopausal patients who have been anovulatory for an extended interval, the endometrium should be biopsied.
2. Biopsy is also recommended before initiation of hormonal therapy for women over age 30 and for those over age 20 who have had prolonged bleeding.
3. Hysteroscopy and endometrial biopsy with a Pipelle aspirator should be done on the first day of menstruation (to avoid an unexpected pregnancy) or anytime if bleeding is continuous. Hysterosonography with uterine saline infusion may also be used.
E. Treatment
1. Medical protocols for anovulatory bleeding (dysfunctional uterine bleeding) are similar to those described above for adolescents.

    2. Hormonal therapy

      a. In women who do not desire immediate fertility, hormonal therapy may be used to treat menorrhagia.

      b. A 21-day package of oral contraceptives is used. The patient should take one pill three times a day for 7 days. During the 7 days of therapy, bleeding should subside, and, following treatment, heavy flow will occur. After 7 days off the hormones, another 21-day package is initiated, taking one pill a day for 21 days, then no pills for 7 days.

      c. Alternatively, medroxyprogesterone (Provera), 10-20 mg per day for days 16 through 25 of each month, will result in a reduction of menstrual blood loss. Pregnancy will not be prevented.

      d. Patients with severe bleeding may have hypotension and tachycardia. These patients require hospitalization, and estrogen (Premarin) should be administered IV as 25 mg q4-6h until bleeding slows (up to a maximum of four doses). Oral contraceptives should be initiated concurrently as described above.

    3. Iron should also be added as ferrous gluconate 325 mg tid.

    4. Surgical treatment can be considered if childbearing is completed and medical management fails to provide relief.

V. Premenopausal, perimenopausal, and postmenopausal years--age 40 and over

A. Anovulatory bleeding accounts for about 90% of abnormal vaginal bleeding in this age group. However, bleeding should be considered to be from cancer until proven otherwise.

B. History, physical examination and laboratory testing are indicated as described above. Menopausal symptoms, personal or family history of malignancy, and use of estrogen should be sought. A pelvic mass requires an evaluation with ultrasonography.

C. Endometrial carcinoma

    1. In a perimenopausal or postmenopausal woman, amenorrhea preceding abnormal bleeding suggests endometrial cancer. Endometrial evaluation is necessary before treatment of abnormal vaginal bleeding.

    2. Before endometrial sampling, determination of endometrial thickness by transvaginal ultrasonography is often useful because biopsy is often not required when the endometrium is less than 5 mm thick.

D. Treatment

    1. Cystic hyperplasia or endometrial hyperplasia without cytologic atypia is treated with depo-medroxyprogesterone, 200 mg IM, then 100 to 200 mg IM every 3 to 4 weeks for 6 to 12 months. Endometrial hyperplasia requires repeat endometrial biopsy every 3 to 6 months.

    2. Atypical hyperplasia requires fractional dilation and curettage, followed by progestin therapy or hysterectomy.

    3. If the patient's endometrium is normal (or atrophic) and contraception is a concern, a low-dose oral contraceptive may be used. If contraception is not needed, estrogen replacement therapy should be prescribed.

    4. Surgical management

      a. Vaginal or abdominal hysterectomy is the most absolute curative treatment.

      b. Dilatation and curettage can be used only as a temporizing measure to stop bleeding.

      c. Endometrial ablation and resection by laser, electrodiathermy "rollerball," or excisional resection are alternatives to hysterectomy.

References: See page 195.

Pelvic Inflammatory Disease

Pelvic inflammatory disease (PID) occurs in one in 10 women during her reproductive years. At least one-fourth of women with PID have serious sequelae, such as infertility, ectopic pregnancy or chronic pelvic pain. PID includes endometritis, salpingitis, tubo-ovarian abscess, and pelvic peritonitis.

I. **Microbiology**
   A. PID is usually polymicrobial, including both aerobic and nonaerobic bacteria. The sexually transmissible organisms most frequently implicated are Neisseria gonorrhoeae and Chlamydia trachomatis.
   B. Mycoplasma hominis and Ureaplasma urealyticum are occasionally isolated. Escherichia coli, streptococcal species, and anaerobes have also been implicated.

II. **Diagnosis**
   A. The diagnosis of PID relies on a high index of suspicion. PID is correctly diagnosed on the basis of clinical and laboratory indicators in only 65% of cases. Therefore, a low threshold for initiating empiric antibiotics is essential.
   B. Risk factors include multiple sex partners, frequent sexual intercourse, and a new sexual partner within the previous 3 months.
   C. PID is characterized by diffuse lower abdominal pain that is often dull and constant, usually bilateral, and less than 2 weeks in duration.
   D. An abnormal vaginal discharge, abnormal bleeding, dysuria, dyspareunia, nausea, vomiting or fever may be present. PID is more likely to begin during the first half of the menstrual cycle.
   E. Abdominal tenderness, adnexal tenderness and cervical motion tenderness are the most frequently observed findings. The presence of symptoms, lower abdominal tenderness, adnexal tenderness, and cervical motion tenderness is sufficient to justify beginning empiric therapy for suspected PID.

Differential Diagnosis of Pelvic Inflammatory Disease	
Appendicitis	Irritable bowel syndrome
Ectopic pregnancy	Somatization
Hemorrhagic ovarian cyst	Gastroenteritis
Ovarian torsion	Cholecystitis
Endometriosis	Nephrolithiasis
Urinary tract Infection	

III. **Laboratory evaluation**
   A. Laboratory studies may be entirely normal. An elevated leukocyte count does not distinguish PID from other diagnoses.
   B. Nonculture tests (eg, Chlamydiazyme, Sure Cell Chlamydia) have good specificity, although sensitivity is less than optimal. Cervical cultures for gonorrhea or Chlamydia require 3-7 days for results and are highly sensitive.
   C. Human immunodeficiency virus (HIV) and syphilis testing are also recommended for patients with suspected PID.
   D. Pelvic ultrasonography can detect pelvic abscesses. Laparoscopy is the "gold standard" for diagnosing PID, and it is recommended when the diagnosis is unclear or when the patient fails to improve.

IV. **Treatment**
   A. **Antibiotic therapy** should be initiated as soon as the diagnosis of PID is suspected, usually before culture results are available.

    B. **CDC guidelines for outpatient treatment of PID**
        1. **Ofloxacin-Metronidazole, Regimen A**
           a. Ofloxacin (Floxin), 400 mg PO bid for 14 days
               Plus
           b. Metronidazole (Flagyl), 500 mg PO bid for 14 days.
        2. **Ceftriaxone-doxycycline, Regimen B**
           a. Ceftriaxone (Rocephin), 250 mg IM (or other parenteral third-generation cephalosporin), or cefoxitin (Mefoxin), 2 gm IM plus probenecid (Benemid), 1 gm PO in a single dose
               Plus
           b. Doxycycline (Vibramycin), 100 mg PO bid for 14 days.
    C. **CDC guidelines for inpatient treatment of PID**
        1. **Cefotetan-doxycycline, Regimen A**
           a. Cefotetan (Cefotan), 2 g IV q12h or cefoxitin (Mefoxin), 2 g IV q6h
               Plus
           b. Doxycycline (Vibramycin), 100 mg IV q12h.
        2. **Clindamycin-gentamicin, Regimen B**
           a. Clindamycin (Cleocin), 900 mg IV q8h
               Plus
           b. Gentamicin (Garamycin), loading dose 2 mg/kg IV , followed by 1.5 mg/kg IV q8h.
        3. Intravenous therapy should be continued for at least 48 hours after clinical improvement. Thereafter, doxycycline, 100 mg PO bid is given for a total of 14 days. If tubo-ovarian abscess is present, clindamycin is used for continued therapy, rather than doxycycline.
        4. The cefoxitin-doxycycline regimen is superior if Chlamydia is suspected as the primary pathogen. The clindamycin-gentamicin regimen has the advantage when more effective anaerobic coverage is desired, such as with tubo-ovarian or pelvic abscesses.
    D. **Partner referral.** Sexual contacts should be treated for GC and Chlamydia, without regard to clinical or laboratory results.

References: See page 195.

Sexually Transmissible Infections

Approximately 12 million patients are diagnosed with a sexually transmissible infection (STI) annually in the United States. Sequella of STIs include infertility, chronic pelvic pain, ectopic pregnancy, and other adverse pregnancy outcomes.

Diagnosis and Treatment of Bacterial Sexually Transmissible Infections			
Organism	Diagnostic Methods	Recommended Treatment	Alternative
Chlamydia trachomatis	Direct fluorescent antibody, enzyme immunoassay, DNA probe, cell culture, DNA amplification	Doxycycline 100 mg PO 2 times a day for 7 days or Azithromycin (Zithromax) 1 g PO	Ofloxacin (Floxin) 300 mg PO 2 times a day for 7 days or erythromycin base 500 mg PO 4 times a day for 7 days or erythromycin ethylsuccinate 800 mg PO 4 times a day for 7 days.

Organism	Diagnostic Methods	Recommended Treatment	Alternative
Neisseria gonorrhoeae	Gram stain of endocervical smear Culture DNA probe	Ceftriaxone (Rocephin) 125 mg IM or Cefixime 400 mg PO or Ciprofloxacin (Cipro) 500 mg PO or Ofloxacin (Floxin) 400 mg PO plus Doxycycline 100 mg 2 times a day for 7 days or azithromycin 1 g PO	Spectinomycin 2 g IM or cephalosporins given as single IM dose of ceftizoxime 500 mg, cefotaxime 500 mg, cefotetan 1 g, and cefoxitin (Mefoxin) 2 g with probenecid 1 g PO; or enoxacin 400 mg PO, lomefloxacin 400 mg PO, or norfloxacin 800 mg PO
Treponema pallidum	Clinical appearance Dark-field microscopy Nontreponemal test: rapid plasma reagin, VDRL Treponemal test: MHA-TP, FTA-ABS	Primary and secondary syphilis and early latent syphilis (<1 year duration): benzathine penicillin G 2.4 million units IM in a single dose.	Penicillin allergy in patients with primary, secondary, or early latent syphilis (<1 year of duration): doxycycline 100 mg PO 2 times a day for 2 weeks.

Diagnosis and Treatment of Viral Sexually Transmissible Infections

Organism	Diagnostic Methods	Recommended Treatment Regimens
Herpes simplex virus	Clinical appearance (confirm with culture) Cell culture	First episode: Acyclovir 400 mg PO 5 times a day for 7-10 days, or famciclovir 250 mg PO 3 times a day for 7-10 days, or valacyclovir 1 g PO 2 times a day for 7-10 days. Recurrent episodes: acyclovir 400 mg PO 3 times a day for 5 days, or 800 mg PO 2 times a day for 5 days or famciclovir 125 mg PO 2 times a day for 5 days, or valacyclovir 500 mg PO 2 times a day for 5 days Daily suppressive therapy: acyclovir 400 mg PO 2 times a day, or famciclovir 250 mg PO 2 times a day, or valacyclovir 250 mg PO 2 times a day, 500 mg PO 1 time a day, or 1000 mg PO 1 time a day
Human papilloma virus	Clinical appearance of condyloma papules Cytology	External warts: Patient may apply podofilox 0.5% solution or gel 2 times a day for 3 days, followed by 4 days of no therapy, for a total of up to 4 cycles, or imiquimod 5% cream at bedtime 3 times a week for up to 16 weeks. Cryotherapy with liquid nitrogen or cryoprobe, repeat every1-2 weeks; or podophyllin, repeat weekly; or TCA 80-90%, repeat weekly if necessary; or surgical removal. Vaginal warts: cryotherapy with liquid nitrogen, or TCA 80-90%, or podophyllin 10-25%

Organism	Diagnostic Methods	Recommended Treatment Regimens
Human immunodeficiency virus	Enzyme immunoassay Western blot (for confirmation) Polymerase chain reaction	Antiretroviral agents

Treatment of Pelvic Inflammatory Disease		
Regimen	Inpatient	Outpatient
A	Cefotetan (Cefotan) 2 g IV q12h; or cefoxitin (Mefoxin) 2 g IV q6h plus doxycycline 100 mg IV or PO q12h.	Ofloxacin (Floxin) 400 mg PO bid for 14 days plus metronidazole 500 mg PO bid for 14 days.
B	Clindamycin 900 mg IV q8h plus gentamicin loading dose IV or IM (2 mg/kg of body weight), followed by a maintenance dose (1.5 mg/kg) q8h.	Ceftriaxone (Rocephin) 250 mg IM once; or cefoxitin 2 g IM plus probenecid 1 g PO; or other parenteral third-generation cephalosporin (eg, ceftizoxime, cefotaxime) plus doxycycline 100 mg PO bid for 14 days.

I. Chlamydia Trachomatis
A. Chlamydia trachomatis is the most prevalent STI in the United States. Chlamydial infections are most common in women age 15-19 years.
B. Routine screening of asymptomatic, sexually active adolescent females undergoing pelvic examination is recommended. Annual screening should be done for women age 20-24 years who are either inconsistent users of barrier contraceptives or who acquired a new sex partner or had more than one sexual partner in the past 3 months.

II. Gonorrhea
A. Gonorrhea has an incidence of 800,000 cases annually. Routine screening for gonorrhea is recommended among women at high risk of infection, including prostitutes, women with a history of repeated episodes of gonorrhea, women under age 25 years with two or more sex partners in the past year, and women with mucopurulent cervicitis.

III. Syphilis
A. Syphilis has an incidence of 100,000 cases annually. The rates are highest in the South, among African Americans, and among those in the 20- to 24-year-old age group.
B. Prostitutes, persons with other STIs, and sexual contacts of persons with active syphilis should be screened.

IV. Herpes simplex virus and human papillomavirus
A. An estimated 200,000-500,000 new cases of herpes simplex occur annually in the United States. New infections are most common in adolescents and young adults.
B. Human papillomavirus affects about 30% of young, sexually active individuals.

V. Human immunodeficiency virus
A. Women account for 19% of adult and adolescent AIDS cases. Eighty-five percent of cases in adult women are among those aged 15-44 years old.

Thirty-eight percent of women were exposed through heterosexual contact.
B. Women at risk for HIV infection include past or present intravenous drug users; those seeking treatment for an STI infection; those exchanging sex for drugs or money or whose sexual partners do; those whose past or present partners were HIV infected, bisexual, or injection drug users; and persons with a history of transfusion between 1978 and 1985.

VI. Pelvic inflammatory disease
A. About 1 million cases of PID occur in the United States annually. Risk factors for PID include young age, low socioeconomic status, unmarried status, residence in an urban area, douching, and smoking. Pelvic inflammatory disease is a polymicrobial infection, but in 65-70% of cases either C trachomatis, N gonorrhoeae, or both are isolated.
B. N gonorrhoeae is usually a symptomatic infection. PID attributable to C trachomatis frequently may be asymptomatic or associated with atypical symptoms such as intermenstrual bleeding or vaginal discharge.

References: See page 195.

Vaginitis

Vaginitis is the most common gynecologic problem encountered by primary care physicians. It may result from bacterial infections, fungal infection, protozoan infection, contact dermatitis, atrophic vaginitis, or allergic reaction.

I. Pathophysiology
A. Vaginitis results from alterations in the vaginal ecosystem, either by the introduction of an organism or by a disturbance that allows normally present pathogens to proliferate.
B. Antibiotics may cause the overgrowth of yeast. Douching may alter the pH level or selectively suppress the growth of endogenous bacteria.

II. Clinical evaluation of vaginal symptoms
A. The type and extent of symptoms, such as itching, discharge, odor, or pelvic pain should be determined.
B. A change in sexual partners or sexual activity, changes in contraception method, medications (antibiotics), and history of prior genital infections should be sought.
C. **Physical examination**
   1. Evaluation of the vagina begins with close inspection of the external genitalia for excoriations, ulcerations, blisters, papillary structures, erythema, edema, mucosal thinning, or mucosal pallor.
   2. The color, texture, and odor of vaginal or cervical discharge should be noted.
D. **Vaginal fluid pH.** The pH level can be determined by placing pH paper on the lateral vaginal wall or immersing the pH paper in the vaginal discharge. A pH level greater than 4.5 often indicates the presence of bacterial vaginosis. It may also indicate the presence of Trichomonas vaginalis.
E. **Saline wet mount**
   1. One swab should be used to obtain a sample from the posterior vaginal fornix, obtaining a "clump" of discharge. Place the sample on a slide, add one drop of normal saline, and apply a coverslip.
   2. Coccoid bacteria and clue cells (bacteria-coated, stippled, epithelial cells) are characteristic of bacterial vaginosis.
   3. Trichomoniasis is confirmed by identification of trichomonads--mobile, oval flagellates. White blood cells are prevalent.
F. **Potassium hydroxide (KOH) preparation**
   1. Place a second sample on a slide, apply one drop of 10% potassium hydroxide (KOH) and a coverslip. A pungent, fishy odor upon addition of KOH--a positive whiff test--strongly indicates bacterial vaginosis.

      2. The KOH prep may reveal Candida in the form of thread-like hyphae and budding yeast.

   G. Screening for STDs. Testing for gonorrhea and chlamydial infection should be completed for women with a new sexual partner, purulent cervical discharge, or cervical motion tenderness.

III. Differential diagnosis

   A. The most common cause of vaginitis is bacterial vaginosis, followed by Candida albicans. The prevalence of trichomoniasis has declined in recent years.

   B. Common nonvaginal etiologies include contact dermatitis from spermicidal creams, latex in condoms, or douching. Any STD can produce vaginal discharge.

Clinical Manifestations of Vaginitis	
Candidal Vaginitis	Nonmalodorous, thick, white, "cottage cheese-like" discharge that adheres to vaginal walls Presence of hyphal forms or budding yeast cells on wet-mount microscopic evaluation Pruritus Normal pH (<4.5)
Bacterial Vaginosis	Thin, dark or dull grey, homogeneous, malodorous discharge that adheres to the vaginal walls Elevated pH level (>4.5) Positive KOH (whiff test) Clue cells on wet-mount microscopic evaluation
Trichomonas Vaginalis	Copious, yellow-gray or green, homogeneous or frothy, malodorous discharge Elevated pH level (>4.5) Mobile, flagellated organisms and leukocytes on wet-mount microscopic evaluation Vulvovaginal irritation, dysuria
Atrophic Vaginitis	Vaginal dryness or burning

IV. Bacterial Vaginosis

   A. Bacterial vaginosis develops when a shift in the normal vaginal ecosystem causes replacement of the usually predominant lactobacilli with mixed bacterial flora. Bacterial vaginosis is the most common type of vaginitis. It is found in 10-25% of patients in gynecologic clinics.

   B. There is usually little itching, no pain, and the symptoms tend to have an indolent course. A malodorous fishy vaginal discharge is characteristic. The odor, a result of anaerobic bacteria, is exacerbated during menses and following intercourse due to the alkaline nature of blood and semen.

   C. There is usually little or no inflammation of the vulva or vaginal epithelium. The vaginal discharge is thin, dark or dull grey, and homogeneous.

   D. A wet-mount will reveal clue cells (epithelial cells stippled with bacteria), an abundance of bacteria of various morphologies, and the absence of homogeneous bacilli (lactobacilli).

   E. Diagnostic criteria (3 of 4 criterial present)
      1. pH >4.0
      2. Clue cells
      3. Positive KOH whiff test
      4. Homogeneous discharge.

F. **Treatment regimens**
   1. **Topical (intravaginal) regimens**
      a. Metronidazole gel (MetroGel) 0.75%, one applicatorful (5 g) bid 5 days.
      b. Clindamycin cream (Cleocin) 2%, one applicatorful (5 g) qhs for 7 nights. Topical therapies have a 90% cure rate.
   2. **Oral metronidazole (Flagyl)**
      a. Oral metronidazole is equally effective as topical therapy. Oral metronidazole has a 90% cure rate.
      b. Dosage is 500 mg bid or 250 mg tid for 7 days. A single 2-g dose is slightly less effective (69-72%) and causes more gastrointestinal upset. All alcohol products should be avoided because nausea and vomiting (disulfiram reaction) may occur.
   3. Routine treatment of sexual partners is not necessary, but it is sometimes helpful for patients with frequent recurrences.
   4. **Persistent cases** should be reevaluated and treatment with clindamycin, 300 mg PO bid for 7 days along with treatment sexual partners.
   5. **Pregnancy.** Clindamycin is recommended, either intravaginally as a daily application of 2% cream or PO, 300 mg bid for 7 days. After the first trimester, oral or topical therapy with metronidazole is acceptable.

V. **Candida Vulvovaginitis**
   A. Candida is the second most common diagnosis associated with vaginal symptoms. It is found in 25% of asymptomatic women. Fungal infections account for 33% of all vaginal infections.
   B. Patients with diabetes mellitus or immunosuppressive conditions such as infection with the human immunodeficiency virus (HIV) are at increased risk for candidal vaginitis. Candidal vaginitis occurs in 25-70% of women after antibiotic therapy.
   C. **Symptoms.** The most common symptom is pruritus. Vulvar burning and an increase or change in consistency of the vaginal discharge may be noted.
   D. **Physical examination**
      1. Candidal vaginitis most often causes a nonmalodorous, thick, adherent, white vaginal discharge that appears "cottage cheese-like."
      2. The vagina is usually hyperemic and edematous. Vulvar erythema may be present.
   E. The normal pH level is not usually altered with candidal vaginitis. Microscopic examination of vaginal discharge diluted with saline (wet-mount) and 10% KOH preparations will reveal hyphal forms or budding yeast cells. Some yeast infections are not detected by microscopy because there are relatively few numbers of organisms.
   F. Confirmation of candidal vaginitis by culture is not recommended. Candida on Pap smear is not a sensitive finding because the yeast is a constituent of the normal vaginal flora.
   G. **Treatment of candida vulvovaginitis**
      1. For severe symptoms and chronic infections, a 7-day course of treatment is used, instead of a 1 day or 3 day course. If there is vulvar involvement, a cream should be used instead of a suppository.
      2. Most C. albicans isolates are susceptible to either clotrimazole or miconazole. An increasing number of nonalbicans Candida species are resistant to the OTC antifungal agents and require the use of prescription antifungal agents. Greater activity has been achieved using terconazole, butoconazole, tioconazole, ketoconazole, and fluconazole.

Antifungal Medications		
Medication	**How Supplied**	**Dosage**
Prescription Agents Oral Agents		
Fluconazole (Diflucan)	150-mg tablet	1 tablet PO 1 time
Ketoconazole (Nizoral)	200 mg	1 tablet PO bid for 5 days
Prescription Topical Agents		
Butoconazole (Femstat)	2% vaginal cream [28 g]	1 vaginally applicatorful qhs for 3 nights
Clotrimazole (Gyne-Lotrimin)	500-mg tablet	1 tablet vaginally qhs 1 time
Miconazole (Monistat 3)	200-mg vaginal suppositories	1 suppository vaginally qhs for 3 nights
Tioconazole (Vagistat)	6.5% cream [5 g]	1 applicatorful vaginally qhs 1 time
Terconazole (Terazol 3)	Cream: 0.4% [45 gm] Cream: 0.8% [20 gm] Vag suppository: 80 mg [3]	One applicatorful intravaginally qhs x 7 days One applicatorful intravaginally qhs x 3 days One suppository intravaginally qhs x 3 days
Over-the-Counter Agents		
Clotrimazole (Gyne-Lotrimin)	1% vaginal cream [45 g] 100-mg vaginal tablets	1 applicatorful vaginally qhs for 7-14 nights 1 tablet vaginally qhs for 7-14 days
Miconazole (Monistat 7)	2% cream [45 g] 100-mg vaginal suppository	1 applicatorful vaginally qhs for 7 days 1 suppository vaginally qhs for 7 days

3. Ketoconazole, 200-mg oral tablets twice daily for 5 days, is effective in treating resistant and recurrent candidal infections. Effectiveness is believed to be a result of the elimination of the rectal reservoir of yeast.
4. Resistant infections also may respond to vaginal use of boric acid, 600 mg in size 0 gelatin capsules daily for 14 days.
5. Treatment of male partners is usually not necessary but may be considered if the partner has yeast balanitis or is uncircumcised.
6. **During pregnancy**, butoconazole (Femstat) should be used in the 2nd or 3rd trimester. Miconazole or clotrimazole may also be used.

H. **Resistant or recurrent cases**
   1. Recurrent infections always should be reevaluated. Repeating topical therapy for a 14-21-day course may be effective. Oral regimens have the potential for eradicating rectal reservoirs.
   2. Cultures are helpful in determining whether a non-candidal and difficult-

to-treat species is present. Patients with recalcitrant disease should be evaluated for diabetes and HIV.

VI. Trichomonas vaginalis

A. Trichomonas, a flagellated anaerobic protozoan, is a sexually transmitted disease with a high transmission rate. Non-sexual transmission is possible because the organism can survive for a few hours in a moist environment.

B. A copious, yellow-gray or green homogeneous discharge is present. A foul odor, vulvovaginal irritation, and, occasionally, dysuria is common. The pH level is usually greater than 4.5.

C. The diagnosis of trichomonal infection is made by examining a wet-mount preparation for mobile, flagellated organisms and an abundance of leukocytes.

D. Occasionally the diagnosis is reported on a Pap test and treatment is recommended.

E. **Treatment of Trichomonas vaginalis**
   1. Metronidazole (Flagyl), 2 g PO in a single dose for both the patient and sexual partner, or 500 mg PO bid for 7 days.
   2. Topical therapy with topical metronidazole is not recommended because the organism may persist in the urethra and Skene's glands after local therapy.
   3. Screening for coexisting sexually transmitted diseases should be completed.
   4. **Recurrent or recalcitrant infections**
      a. If patients are compliant but develop recurrent infections, treatment of their sexual partners should be confirmed.
      b. Cultures should be performed. In patients with persistent infection, a resistant trichomonad strain may require high dosages of metronidazole 2.5 g/d, often combined with intravaginal metronidazole for 10 days.

VII. Other diagnoses causing vaginal symptoms

A. One-third of patients with vaginal symptoms will not have laboratory evidence of bacterial vaginosis, Candida, or Trichomonas.

B. Other causes of the vaginal symptoms include cervicitis, allergic reactions, and vulvodynia.

C. **Atrophic vaginitis** should be considered in postmenopausal patients if the mucosa appears pale and thin and wet-mount findings are negative.
   1. Oral estrogen (Premarin) 0.625 mg qd should provide relief.
   2. Estradiol vaginal cream 0.01% may be effective as 2-4 g daily for 1-2 weeks, then 1 g one to three times weekly.
   3. Conjugated estrogen vaginal cream may be effective as 2-4 g daily (3 weeks on, 1 week off) for 3-6 months.

D. **Allergy and chemical irritation**
   1. Patients should be questioned about use of substances that cause allergic or chemical irritation, such as deodorant soaps, laundry detergent, vaginal contraceptives, bath oils, perfumed or dyed toilet paper, hot tub or swimming pool chemicals, and synthetic clothing.
   2. Topical steroids and systemic antihistamines can help alleviate the symptoms until the irritant can be identified.

References: See page 195.

Urinary Incontinence

Urinary incontinence is defined as the involuntary loss of urine. Incontinence is 2-3 times more common among women than men, and is primarily related to childbirth and menopause. Urinary incontinence affects 15-30% of women older than the age of 60 and more than 50% of nursing home residents.

I. Classification of urinary incontinence

A. **Stress incontinence** is characterized by involuntary loss of urine occurring with increases in intra-abdominal pressure. Women complain of urinary leakage with cough, exercise, laughing, and Valsalva maneuver. Stress incontinence is caused by urethral hypermobility or intrinsic sphincter deficiency. Urethral hypermobility, the most common cause of stress incontinence, occurs when there is loss of the anatomic support of the bladder neck. This damage to the bladder neck supports may be the result of vaginal delivery or tissue atrophy, resulting from advancing age and estrogen withdrawal. Intrinsic sphincter deficiency is caused by decreased urethral resting tone. Stress incontinence can occur with advanced pelvic prolapse.

B. **Detrusor instability (urge incontinence)** is defined as the involuntary loss of urine associated with a sudden and strong desire to void (urgency). Spontaneous uninhibited detrusor overactivity results in detrusor contractions. Patients with this condition complain of an inability to control voiding and experience a sudden urgency to void, which is sometimes unsuppressible. These patients report urinary frequency (>7 times/day), nocturia (>1 time/night), enuresis, and pelvic pain. Although detrusor instability is most often iatrogenic, secondary causes include urinary tract infection, anti-incontinence surgery, bladder stones or foreign bodies, and bladder cancer.

Reversible Causes and Risk Factors for Urinary Incontinence

• Immobility/chronic degenerative disease	• Environmental barriers
• Impaired cognition	• High-impact physical activities
• Medications	• Diabetes
• Morbid obesity	• Stroke
• Diuretics	• Estrogen deprivation
• Smoking	• Pelvic muscle weakness
• Fecal impaction	• Childhood nocturnal enuresis
• Delirium	• Race
• Low fluid intake	• Pregnancy/vaginal delivery/episiotomy

Medications Causing Incontinence

Enalapril	Hyoscyamine
Benztropine	Oxybutynin
Trihexyphenidyl	Prazosin
Benzodiazepines	Terazosin
Cisapride	Thioridazine
Furosemide	Chlorpromazine
Hydrochlorothiazide	Haloperidol
Alcohol	Clozapine

II. Clinical evaluation of urinary incontinence

A. **Duration, characteristics, and severity** of the incontinence, precipitating factors and reversible causes should be assessed. Dysuria, urgency, pelvic pain, dyspareunia, constipation, fecal incontinence, pelvic prolapse, or abnormal vaginal discharge should be sought. A history of diabetes, thyroid disease, spinal cord injury, cerebral vascular accidents, urethral sphincter damage, or fistula conditions should be excluded.

B. **Estrogen status** should be determined because hypoestrogenism can contribute to recurrent cystitis, detrusor instability, and stress incontinence. Patients should be questioned about recurrent urinary tract infections, kidney stones, bladder pain, or hematuria.

C. **Physical examination**
1. **Neurologic examination.** Normal sensation in the perineal and the back of the leg confirms intact sensory enervation of the lower urinary tract. Sacral reflex activity is tested via the anal reflex-stroking the skin with a cotton swab adjacent to the anus causes reflex contraction of the external anal sphincter. Pelvic floor muscle tone can be assessed by voluntary contraction of the anal sphincter and vagina during a bimanual exam.
2. **Pelvic exam** should be performed to assess the external genitalia, perineal sensation, presence of pelvic organ prolapse (cystocele, enterocele, rectocele, uterine prolapse), estrogen status, and pelvic muscle strength. A bimanual exam with rectovaginal exam should be done to rule out pelvic masses.
3. **Observation of urine loss** while the patient has a full bladder can be performed by having the patient cough vigorously in the standing position. If instantaneous leakage occurs with cough, stress urinary incontinence is likely while detrusor instability (urge incontinence) is suggested by delayed or sustained leakage.
4. **Urethral hypermobility** due to loss of bladder neck support can be assessed using a cotton swab test. A sterile, lubricated cotton swab is inserted transurethrally into the bladder and then withdrawn slowly until resistance is felt, then the patient is then asked to cough or perform a Valsalva maneuver. A $30°$ deflection indicates urethral hypermobility.

D. **Post-void residual** is useful to rule out overflow incontinence and incomplete bladder emptying, and a urinalysis and/or urine culture to rule out urinary tract infection. After a normal void, a post-void residual urine volume is determined using a catheterization or bladder scan. A post-void residual should be less than below 100 cc.

E. **Cystometry** is used to measure the pressure volume relationship of the bladder as it distends. Complex cystometry uses specialized equipment with pressure catheters to record bladder pressures. Simple cystometry can readily be performed in the office with a red rubber catheter, a syringe, and sterile water.

F. **Urinalysis or urine culture** should be obtained. Creatinine BUN, glucose, and calcium are recommended if compromised renal function is suspected or if polyuria is present.

III. **Treatment of urinary incontinence**
A. **Detrusor instability (urge incontinence)** is treated with bladder retraining and pharmacologic therapy.
B. **Stress incontinence** is treated with Kegel exercises, pharmacotherapy, biofeedback, electrical stimulation, medical devices, or surgery.
C. **Behavioral modification**
1. Detrusor instability (urge incontinence) may respond to dietary restriction of caffeine, alcohol, chocolate, and spicy food, as these can all cause bladder irritation. Scheduled toileting should be offered to incontinent patients. Bladder training (timed voiding) helps to progressively distend the bladder and allows the patient to regain control over voiding patterns. The patient is instructed to void at pre-assigned times during the waking hours. The initial voiding interval is set at less than the current voiding interval and is gradually increased.
2. **Kegel's exercise.** Pelvic muscle exercises are used in stress urinary incontinence and detrusor instability (urge incontinence). A typical regimen of pelvic floor exercises is based on sets of contractions of the levator muscles performed 2-4 times daily. This regimen results in a 60-

70% improvement in their symptoms.
- **D. Pharmacotherapy**
  1. Pharmacotherapy is used for detrusor instability (urge incontinence) and stress urinary incontinence.
  2. **Oxybutynin (Ditropan)** is the agent of choice (2.5-5 mg PO tid-qid). Start patients on 2.5 mg po bid and then titrate up based on symptoms. The primary side effects of anticholinergic medications include dry mouth, constipation, blurred vision, change in mental status, and nausea. These medications are contraindicated in patients with narrow angle glaucoma. Other anticholinergic agents, including propantheline, dicyclomine, and flavoxate, may be used in patients with a poor response to oxybutynin.
  3. **Tolterodine (Detrol)** is a bladder selective anticholinergic agent that is associated with improved symptoms and reduced side effects.
  4. **Imipramine (Tofranil)** has been shown to be effective in the treatment of both stress and detrusor instability (urge incontinence). Dosage is 25-100 mg daily. Side effects include orthostatic hypertension and dry mouth.
  5. **Alpha-adrenergic agonists,** phenylpropanolamine (PPA) and pseudoephedrine are useful in the treatment of stress incontinence. Dosage for PPA is 25-100 mg PO in a sustained release form (bid) and for pseudoephedrine, 15-30 mg PO tid.
  6. **Estrogen replacement,** either oral or vaginal, should be used as an adjunctive agent for postmenopausal women with stress urinary incontinence. The combination of an alpha-agonist and estrogen have a synergistic effect. Progestin should be added in patients who have a uterus.

Pharmacologic Agents for the Treatment of Urinary Incontinence			
Medication	Dosage	Mechanism of Action	Indication
Oxybutynin (Ditropan)	2.5 mg bid-5 mg tid	Anticholinergic/Spasmolytic	Detrusor instability
Hyoscyamine (Levsin, Cystospaz)	0.15 mg tid-qid 0.375 mg bid-tid (extended release)	Anticholinergic	Detrusor instability
Flavoxilate (Urispas)	100-200 mg tid-qid	Anticholinergic/Spasmolytic	Detrusor instability
Tolterodine (Detrol)	2 mg bid	Anticholinergic	Detrusor instability
Propantheline bromide (Pro-Banthine)	7.5 mg tid	Anticholinergic	Detrusor instability
Phenylpropanolamine (Entex)	5 mg bid	Alpha-adrenergic stimulation	Stress incontinence
Pseudoephedrine (Sudafed)	60 mg qid	Alpha-adrenergic stimulation	Stress incontinence

Medication	Dosage	Mechanism of Action	Indication
Imipramine (Tofranil)	25-75 mg daily	Anticholinergic and alpha-adrenergic stimulation	Detrusor instability Stress incontinence
Estrogen (Premarin)	0.625 mg po or vaginally, daily	Beneficial effects on urethral mucosa and sphincter	Detrusor instability Stress incontinence

E. **Surgical correction**
1. Surgery is used primarily in the treatment of stress urinary incontinence due to urethral hypermobility or intrinsic sphincter deficiency. Urethral hypermobility is corrected with retropubic urethropexy, transvaginal needle suspension, or a suburethral sling.
2. **Retropubic urethropexy:** vaginal tissue underneath the urethra is suspended to the pubic symphysis (Marshall-Marchetti-Krantz urethropexy) or Cooper's ligament (Burch colposuspension). The transvaginal needle suspension procedure is performed via the vaginal route with a small abdominal incision. The success rates for the retropubic urethropexy, transvaginal needle suspension, and suburethral sling are 80%, 70%, and 85%, respectively.
3. Intrinsic sphincter deficiency can be managed with a suburethral sling or periurethral collagen injections.

References: See page 195.

Pubic Infections

I. **Human Papilloma Virus**
   A. HPV is the most common tumor of the vulva. The incubation period varies from weeks to months.
   B. Condyloma acuminata lesions appear as rough, verrucous papillomas on the genitalia. Enlargement often occurs during pregnancy and sometimes lesions disappear spontaneously. No screening tests for subclinical infection exist. Pap smear diagnosis of HPV does not correlate well with detection of HPV DNA.
   C. **Treatment of genital/perianal warts**
      1. **Cryosurgery with liquid nitrogen or cryoprobe** is more effective than topical therapies. Lesions should be frozen until a 2 mm margin of freeze appears, then allowed to thaw, then refrozen. Repeat freeze several times.
      2. **Podophyllin** 25% in of benzoin may be applied and washed off 4 hours later. Two or 3 applications, 1 week apart, may be needed. Podophyllin should not be used on the vagina or cervix; it is contraindicated in pregnancy.
      3. **Trichloracetic acid (80%).** Apply to lesion with a cotton-tip applicator, then observe for 5-10 minutes; 2 or 3 applications may be needed, 1 week apart. Burning is common. TCA can be used on the cervix, vagina, and external warts; it can be used during pregnancy.
      4. **Podofilox 0.5% (Condylox)** solution for self-treatment: Apply twice daily for 3 days followed by 4 days of no therapy. This cycle may be repeated as necessary for a total of 4 cycles; not for use on vagina or cervix.

     5. Surgical excision and electrocoagulation or laser may be used.
     6. Large, bulky or extensive lesions
       a. General anesthesia and wire loop cautery is effective.
       b. Topical 5-fluorouracil cream in a 1-2% concentration is effective in the treatment of vaginal condylomata.
     7. Recurrence rates are high (25% within 3 months). No therapy has been proven to eradicate HPV.
  D. Partner referral
     1. Examination is usually not required. The use of condoms may reduce transmission to partners.
     2. Annual Pap smears are recommended

II. Molluscum Contagiosum
  A. This disease is produced by a virus of the pox virus family and is spread by sexual or close personal contact. Lesions are usually asymptomatic and multiple, with a central umbilication. Lesions can be spread by autoinoculation and last from 6 months to many years.
  B. Diagnosis. The characteristic appearance is adequate for diagnosis, but biopsy may be used to confirm the diagnosis.
  C. Treatment. Lesions are removed by sharp dermal curette, liquid nitrogen cryosurgery, or electrodesiccation.

III. Pediculosis Pubis (Crabs)
  A. Clinical features
     1. Phthirus pubis is a blood sucking louse that is unable to survive more than 24 hours off the body. It is often transmitted sexually and is principally found on the pubic hairs.
     2. Diagnosis is confirmed by locating nits or adult lice on the hair shafts.
  B. Treatment
     1. Permethrin cream (Elimite), 5% is the most effective treatment; it is applied for 10 minutes and washed off.
     2. Kwell shampoo, lathered for at least 4 minutes, can also be used, but it is contraindicated in pregnancy or lactation.
     3. All contaminated clothing and linen should be laundered.

IV. Pubic Scabies
  A. This highly contagious infestation is caused by the Sarcoptes scabiei (0.2-0.4 mm in length). The infestation is transmitted by intimate contact or by contact with infested clothing.
     1. The female mite burrows into the skin, and after 1 month, severe pruritus develops A multiform eruption may develop, characterized by papules, vesicles, pustules, urticarial wheals, and secondary infections on the hands, wrists, elbows, belt line, buttocks, genitalia, and outer feet.
  B. Diagnosis is confirmed by visualization of burrows and observation of parasites, eggs, larvae, or red fecal compactions under microscopy.
  C. Treatment. Permethrin 5% cream (Elimite) is massaged in from the neck down and remove by washing after 8 hours.

References: See page 195.

Urologic Disorders

Benign Prostatic Hyperplasia

The prostate normally grows larger as men age. After age 40, benign prostatic hyperplasia commonly develops. BPH affects half of men by age 60, and at least 80% by age 80. BPH is not a precursor or predisposing factor to prostate cancer. Symptoms include urinary stream weakness, hesitancy, urgency, nocturia, incomplete bladder emptying, retention, and straining.

I. **Pathophysiology**
   A. Prostatic stromal tissue is controlled by the adrenergic nervous system. Alpha-1 receptors control 80% of the activity of prostatic smooth muscle cells, causing contraction of the prostate.
   B. Many men with palpably enlarged prostates are not symptomatic, while some patients with small prostates have significant voiding symptoms or urinary retention.
   C. Obstruction forces the bladder to generate higher pressures than normal to achieve micturition. Increased muscle mass in the bladder leads to reduced bladder elasticity and compliance, which manifests as a reduction in bladder capacity.
   D. If the obstruction is not relieved, bladder failure will result. This process produces the classic obstructive voiding symptoms of hesitancy, intermittency, decreased force of the stream, postvoid dribbling, and a feeling of incomplete bladder emptying.

II. **Clinical evaluation of benign prostatic hypertrophy**
   A. Symptoms of BPH may be obstructive, which are secondary to bladder outlet obstruction or impaired bladder contractility, or irritative, which result from decreased vesicle compliance and increased bladder instability.

Symptoms of Benign Prostatic Hyperplasia	
Irritative Symptoms	**Obstructive Symptoms**
Nocturia	Decreased force of stream
Urinary frequency	Urinary hesitancy
Urinary urgency	Terminal dribbling
Dysuria	Straining to urinate
Urge incontinence	Prolonged voiding
Small voided volume	Retention
	Overflow incontinence

   B. **Obstructive symptoms** include a weak stream, hesitancy, abdominal straining, terminal dribbling, an intermittent stream, and retention; frequency, nocturia, urgency, and pain during urination are common.
   C. **Physical examination**
      1. A digital rectal examination should search for nodules and induration or irregularities. A focused neurologic examination should rule out a neurologic cause of symptoms.
      2. Prostate cancer is suggested by a prostate nodule or a hardened area of the prostate on the digital rectal examination.
   D. **Laboratory assessment.** Urinalysis and a serum creatinine assay are useful to ascertain there is no infection, hematuria, or decreased renal function. Measurement of PSA to detect prostate cancer is optional.
   E. **Differential diagnosis**
      1. The symptoms of BPH are not specific for prostate cancer because symptomatic and asymptomatic older men have the same rate of

prostate cancer.
2. Diabetes mellitus is the most common nonobstructive cause of obstructive voiding symptoms is Diabetes leads to peripheral neuropathy and detrusor muscle failure. Glucose will be present on the urinalysis.
3. **Urinary tract infection** can mimic the irritative symptoms of BPH; however, pyuria will be present on urinalysis.
4. **Drugs that exacerbate prostatism** include alcohol, caffeine, anticholinergic agents, first-generation antihistamines, tricyclic antidepressants, and urinary anti-spasmodic agents.

F. **Complications of benign prostatic hypertrophy**
   1. **Urinary tract infection** can be recurrent or cause sepsis.
   2. **Severe obstruction and hydronephrosis** may cause uremia manifest by malaise and nausea.
   3. **Urinary retention** (200 to 300 mL post-voided residual urine) may present as abdominal pain or suprapubic fullness.

III. Treatment of benign prostatic hyperplasia

A. If symptoms are mild, watchful waiting is recommended. Patients with moderate symptoms should begin medical treatment. Severe symptoms may warrant initiation of medical treatment, but eventually surgical intervention will be required.

B. **Alpha-1-adrenergic receptor blockers**
   1. Alpha-1 blockers relax the smooth muscle of the prostate. Alpha-blockers are the drugs of choice for BPH because they are effective and because they begin to work immediately. Men with hypertension and benign prostatic hypertrophy may be able to control both problems with only one medication. Terazosin and doxazosin are long-acting alpha-1-blockers.
   2. **Terazosin (Hytrin)** is initiated with a dosage of 1 mg qhs, and then raised to 2 mg, 5 mg, and 10 mg if necessary; a response may not be seen for 4-6 weeks.
   3. **Doxazosin (Cardura)** is given at a dosage of 0.5 mg qd.
   4. The main side effects of alpha-blockers are dizziness (10%), fatigue (7%), and postural hypotension (7%). The incidence and severity of these side effects can be decreased by bedtime administration.
   5. Alpha blockers are more effective in relieving symptoms than finasteride.

C. **Hormonal manipulation. Finasteride (Proscar)** is an antiandrogen and 5-alpha reductase inhibitor that blocks prostatic conversion of testosterone to dihydrotestosterone, resulting in prostate shrinkage. Finasteride (5 mg per day) requires 3-6 months to produce results, and only 33-50% report improvement. It is used primarily for men with significant cardiac disease who can not tolerate alpha-1 blockers. Adverse effects include decreased libido and impotence.

IV. Surgical therapy

A. **Transurethral resection of the prostate**
   1. TURP is the most effective way to relieve symptoms of prostatism. Good resolution of urinary symptoms is achieved in 80-90%.
   2. The total morbidity from TURP is about 18%; impotence occurs in 10%. Incontinence occurs in 3% and 1% die.
   3. **Definite indications for surgery.** Urinary retention, increased creatinine, recurrent urinary tract infections, and bladder stones.
   4. **Relative indications for surgery:** Recurrent gross hematuria, severe symptoms.

References: See page 195.

Prostatitis and Prostatodynia

I. **Acute bacterial prostatitis**
   A. Acute bacterial prostatitis is characterized by abrupt onset of fever and chills with symptoms of urinary tract infection or obstruction, low back or perineal pain, malaise, arthralgia, and myalgias. Urinary retention may develop.
   B. **Physical exam.** The prostate is enlarged, indurated, very tender, and warm. Prostate massage is contraindicated because it may cause bacterial dissemination.
   C. **Laboratory evaluation**
      1. Urine reveals WBC's. Culture reveals gram-negative organisms such as E coli or other Enterobacteriaceae.
      2. Nosocomial infections are often associated with a Foley catheter and may be caused by Pseudomonas, enterococci, or S. aureus.
   D. **Treatment** of acute prostatitis requires 28 days of antibiotic treatment. Fluoroquinolones are the drugs of choice.
      1. Ciprofloxacin (Cipro) 500 mg PO bid.
      2. Norfloxacin (Noroxin) 400 mg PO bid.
      3. Ofloxacin (Floxin) 400 mg PO/IV bid.
      4. Trimethoprim/SMX (TMP-SMX, Septra) 160/800 mg (1 DS tab) PO bid.
      5. Doxycycline (Vibramycin) 100 mg PO bid.
   E. **Extremely ill septic patients with high fever**
      1. Hospitalization for bed rest, hydration, analgesics, antipyretics, stool softeners.
      2. Ampicillin 1 gm IV q4-6h **AND** Gentamicin or tobramycin - loading dose of 100-120 mg IV (1.5-2 mg/kg); then 80 mg-1 mg/kg IV q8h (2-5 mg/kg/d) **OR**
      3. Ciprofloxacin (Cipro) 200 mg IV q12h.

II. **Chronic bacterial prostatitis**
   A. Chronic prostatitis is characterized by recurrent urinary tract infections, perineal, low back or suprapubic pain, testicular, or penile pain, voiding dysfunction, post-ejaculatory pain, and intermittent hematospermia.
   B. **Exam.** The prostate is usually normal and nontender, but it may occasionally be enlarged and tender.
   C. **Laboratory evaluation**
      1. Urinalysis and culture usually shows low grade bacteriuria (E. coli or other Gram negative Enterobacteriaceae, Enterococcus faecalis, S. aureus, coagulase negative staphylococcus).
      2. Microscopic examination of expressed prostatic secretions reveals more than 10-15 WBCs per high-power field.
   D. **Long-term treatment (16 weeks)**
      1. A fluoroquinolone is the drug of choice.
      2. Ciprofloxacin (Cipro) 250-500 mg PO bid.
      3. Ofloxacin (Floxin) 200-400 mg PO/IV bid.
      4. Trimethoprim/sulfamethoxazole (TMP-SMZ, Septra) 160/800 mg (1 DS tab) PO bid.
      5. **Suppression** is indicated if recurrent symptomatic infections occur: Fluoroquinolone or TMP/SMX (1 single-strength tab qd).

III. **Chronic nonbacterial prostatitis**
   A. The most common type of prostatitis is nonbacterial. It is eight times more frequent than bacterial prostatitis. It is characterized by perineal, suprapubic or low back pain, and irritative or obstructive urinary symptoms. Symptoms and exam are similar to chronic bacterial prostatitis but with no recurrent UTI history.
   B. Cultures are sterile and show no bacteria or uropathogens. Microscopic examination reveals 10-15 WBC's per high-power field.

C. **Treatment (2-4 week trial of antibiotics):**
   1. Doxycycline (100 mg bid) or erythromycin (500 mg qid) may relieve symptoms.
   2. Irritative symptoms may respond to nonsteroidal anti-inflammatory agents, muscle relaxants, anticholinergics, hot sitz baths, normal sexual activity, regular mild exercise, and avoidance of spicy foods and excessive caffeine and alcohol. Serial prostatic massage may be helpful.
   3. The disorder is usually self-limited. In persistent cases, carcinoma of the prostate and interstitial cystitis must be excluded.

IV. Prostatodynia
A. Symptoms are similar to prostatitis, but there are no objective findings suggesting that symptoms arise in the prostate gland. Age ranges between 22-56 years.
B. Symptoms include pain or discomfort in the perineum, groin, testicles, penis and urethra. Irritative or obstructive voiding symptoms are predominant. Stress and emotional problems are often contributing factors. Tender musculature may be found on rectal examination.
C. **Urine** is normal (no WBC or bacteria), sterile for uropathogen, and urodynamic testing may detect uncoordinated voiding patterns. Cystoscopic examination may be useful.
D. **Treatment**
   1. Alpha-adrenergic blocking agents (terazosin 1-5 mg qd, and doxazosin 1-4 mg qd) can be used to relax the bladder neck sphincter. Muscle-relaxing agents such as diazepam (Valium 2-10 mg bid) may provide relief.
   2. Nonsteroidal anti-inflammatory agents, sitz baths, normal sexual activity, avoidance of stress, spicy foods, caffeine, and alcohol may be beneficial.

References: See page 195.

Acute Epididymoorchitis

I. Clinical evaluation of testicular pain
A. Epididymoorchitis is indicated by a unilateral painful testicle and a history of unprotected intercourse, new sexual partner, urinary tract infection, dysuria, or discharge. Symptoms may occur following acute lifting or straining.
B. The epididymis and testicle are painful, swollen, and tender. The scrotum may be erythematosus and warm, with associated spermatic cord thickening or penile discharge.
C. **Differential diagnosis of painful scrotal swelling**
   1. Epididymitis, testicular torsion, testicular tumor, hernia.
   2. Torsion is characterized by sudden onset, age <20, an elevated testicle, and previous episodes scrotal pain. The epididymis is usually located anteriorly on either side, and there is an absence of evidence of urethritis and UTI.
   3. Epididymitis is favored by fever, laboratory evidence of urethritis or cystitis, and increased scrotal warmth.

II. Laboratory evaluation of epididymoorchitis
A. Epididymoorchitis is indicated by leukocytosis with a left shift; UA shows pyuria and bacteriuria. Midstream urine culture will reveal gram negative bacilli. Chlamydia and Neisseria cultures should be taken.
B. **Common pathogens**
   1. **Younger men.** Epididymoorchitis is usually associated with sexually transmitted organisms such as Chlamydia and gonorrhea.
   2. **Older men.** Epididymoorchitis is usually associated with a concomitant urinary tract infection or prostatitis caused by E. coli, proteus, Klebsiella,

Enterobacter, or Pseudomonas.

III. Treatment of epididymoorchitis
A. Bed rest, scrotal elevation with athletic supporter, an ice pack, analgesics, and antipyretics are prescribed. Sexual and physical activity should be avoided.
B. **Sexually transmitted epididymitis in sexually active males**
  1. Ceftriaxone (Rocephin) 250 mg IM x 1 dose **AND** doxycycline 100 mg PO bid x 10 days **OR**
  2. Ofloxacin (Floxin) 300 mg bid x 10 days.
  3. Treat sexual partners
C. **Epididymitis secondary to urinary tract infection**
  1. TMP/SMX DS bid for 10 days or ofloxacin (Floxin) 300 mg PO bid for 10 days. **OR**
  2. Ofloxacin (Floxin) 300 mg po bid for 10 days **AND** doxycycline 100 gm PO bid x 10 days.

References: See page 195.

Erectile Dysfunction

Age is the single most important variable associated with erectile difficulty. About 20-30 million American men are impotent. Parasympathetic fibers are the primary neuronal system involved in the erectile process. Adrenergic stimulation results in penile detumescence. Noncholinergic, nonadrenergic neurons in the penis cause penile tumescence through release of nitric oxide. Adequate androgen (testosterone) levels are usually required for libido.

I. Evaluation of erectile dysfunction
A. Social or psychological factors should be evaluated. Medical conditions, medications, and history of prior pelvic surgical procedures should be sought. Physical examination should search for abnormalities of sexual characteristics or of the genitalia. Evidence of trauma, plaques, or testicular abnormalities should be assessed. A neurologic examination should be performed.
B. **Laboratory work-up.** Complete blood count and chemistries should be obtained. Serum testosterone measurement is recommended in all impotent patients over age 50. In patients younger than 50 years, serum testosterone determination is recommended only in cases of low sexual desire or abnormal physical findings. Serum prolactin should be measured in patients with low sexual desire, gynecomastia, and/or testosterone less than 4 ng/mL.

II. Treatment of erectile dysfunction
A. **Testosterone cypionate** (200 mg IM q 2 weeks) or testosterone patches may be beneficial if the serum-free testosterone is low (<9 ng/dL). Older males (>50 years) are at risk for development of prostate cancer. A careful rectal examination and PSA testing is recommended prior to institution of, and during, testosterone therapy. Patients with elevated prolactin and a pituitary secreting tumor should be referred to an endocrinologist or neurosurgeon for bromocriptine treatment or surgical ablation.
B. **Sildenafil (Viagra)** is the only oral medication available for erectile dysfunction. A type-5-phosphodiesterase inhibitor, the drug potentiates the effects of nitrous oxide on sinusoidal smooth muscle. It comes in 25, 50, and 100 mg tablets which should be taken about 1-1.5 hours prior to intercourse. Initial dose is 50 mg at a maximum frequency of one per day. The dose can be increased up to 100 mg. The drug can potentiate the hypotensive effects of nitrates; therefore, nitrate us is an absolute contraindication. Adverse reactions include headache and changes in vision. Other oral medications awaiting FDA approval include phentolamine

(Vasomax) and apomorphine.

C. **Vacuum constriction devices (VCD)** are an effective treatment alternative for erectile dysfunction. The design involves a plastic cylinder that is placed on the penis with negative pressure created. A constriction band is placed at the base of the penis. Almost every patient can be a candidate for these devices. Contraindications include penile angulation deformity, prior history of priapism, and patients taking anticoagulants.

D. **Pharmacologic injection therapies** include papaverine, phentolamine, and prostaglandin E-1 (PGE-1), either as single agents or in combination therapy. The only FDA-approved medications for injection are Caverject and Edex.

E. **Intraurethral prostaglandin suppositories (MUSE),** have the advantage that penile injection is not necessary. MUSE comes in four dosages- 125, 250, 500, and 1000 mcg. A condom should be used for intercourse with a pregnant female. The response rate of is 40-60%.

F. **Surgical treatment** of erectile dysfunction consists of placement of a penile prosthesis. This therapy should only be considered if all other options have been explored. Devices available include semirigid or inflatable prostheses. An occasionally indicated treatment option is vascular surgery.

References: See page 195.

Psychiatric Disorders

Depression

Depression has a 6-month prevalence of 5.8 percent and a lifetime prevalence of 17%. Three fourths of patients with depression improve with therapy.

I. Diagnosis
   A. Clinical evaluation should identify characteristics of depressed mood, loss of interest in usually pleasurable activities, and history of past depression. Insomnia, hallucinations, suicidal ideation and planning, or alcohol and drug abuse should be sought. Symptoms may also include guilt feelings, thoughts of worthlessness, energy changes/fatigue, concentration/attention impairment, and appetite/weight changes.
   B. Family history may reveal depression, suicide, or drug or alcohol abuse.
   C. Suicide risk. The risk of suicide is higher in depressed patients who are divorced or widowed, elderly, white, male or living alone, and in those with chronic medical illness or psychotic symptoms.

Diagnostic Criteria for Major Depression, DSM IV

Cluster 1: Physical or neurovegetative symptoms
Sleep disturbance
Appetite/weight changes
Attention/concentration problem
Energy-level change/fatigue
Psychomotor disturbance

Cluster 2: Psychologic or psychosocial symptoms
Depressed mood and/or
Interest/pleasure reduction
Guilt feelings
Suicidal thoughts

Note: Diagnosis of major depression requires at least one of the first two symptoms under cluster 2 and four of the remaining symptoms to be present for at least two weeks. Symptoms should not be accounted for by bereavement.

II. Laboratory evaluation may include a complete blood cell count, chemistry panel, thyroid stimulating hormone, and glucose. An electrocardiogram is recommended if the patient is more than 40 years of age.
III. Treatment of depression
   A. Since all antidepressants are effective, selection of a drug is based on considerations of safety, tolerability, cost, and convenience of dosing.
   B. Selective serotonin reuptake inhibitors
      1. Drugs of choice for the treatment of major depressive disorder are the selective serotonin reuptake inhibitors (SSRIs), fluoxetine (Prozac), paroxetine (Paxil), and sertraline (Zoloft), because they have favorable safety profiles and are easy to administer. They are not lethal in overdose, and patients are less likely to discontinue treatment because of adverse effects.
      2. Side effects of SSRIs. Nausea, common during the first week, tends to wane as the patient develops tolerance. Fluvoxamine (LuVox) may

cause less nausea. Insomnia can be a problem with SSRIs; therefore, these activating antidepressants are usually administered in the morning.

3. Patients taking sertraline and paroxetine might experience considerable improvement in sexual function with scheduled weekend drug holidays. Anorgasmia may be managed by dosage reduction, treatment with cyproheptadine, or prescribing a different antidepressant, such as bupropion (Wellbutrin).

Characteristics of Common Antidepressants

Drug	Recommended Dosage	Comments
Selective Serotonin Reuptake Inhibitors (SSRIs)		
Fluoxetine (Prozac)	10-20 mg/d initially, taken in AM	Common side effects: Anxiety, insomnia, agitation, nausea, anorgasmia, erectile dysfunction, headache, anorexia.
Fluvoxamine (LuVox)	50-100 mg qhs; max 300 mg/d [50, 100 mg]	Headache, nausea, sedation, abnormal ejaculation, diarrhea
Paroxetine (Paxil)	20 mg/d initially, given in AM; increase in 10-mg/d increments as needed to max of 50 mg/d. [10, 20, 30, 40 mg]	Headache, nausea, somnolence, dizziness, insomnia, abnormal ejaculation, anxiety, diarrhea, dry mouth.
Sertraline (Zoloft)	50 mg/d, increasing as needed to max of 200 mg/d [50, 100 mg]	Insomnia, agitation, dry mouth, headache, nausea, anorexia, sexual dysfunction.
Secondary Amine Tricyclic Antidepressants		
Desipramine (Norpramin, generics)	100-200 mg/d, gradually increasing to 300 mg/d as tolerated.[10, 25, 50, 75, 100, 150 mg]	No sedation; may have stimulant effect; best taken in morning to avoid insomnia.
Nortriptyline (Pamelor)	25 mg tid-qid, max 150 mg/d. [10, 25, 50, 75 mg]	Sedating
Tertiary Amine Tricyclics		
Amitriptyline (Elavil, generics)	75 mg/d qhs-bid, increasing to 150-200 mg/d. [25, 50, 75, 100, 150 mg]	Sedative effect precedes antidepressant effect. High anticholinergic activity.
Clomipramine (Anafranil)	25 mg/d, increasing gradually to 100 mg/d; max 250 mg/d; may be given once qhs [25, 50, 75 mg].	Relatively high sedation, anticholinergic activity, and seizure risk.
Protriptyline (Vivactil)	5-10 mg PO tid-qid; 15-60 mg/d [5, 10 mg]	Useful in anxious depression; nonsedating

Drug	Recommended Dosage	Comments
Doxepin (Sinequan, generics)	50-75 mg/d, increasing up to 150-300 mg/d as needed [10, 25, 50, 75, 100, 150 mg]	Sedating. Also indicated for anxiety. Contraindicated in patients with glaucoma or urinary retention.
Imipramine (Tofranil, generics)	75 mg/d in a single dose qhs, increasing to 150 mg/d; 300 mg/d. [10, 25, 50 mg]	High sedation and anticholinergic activity. Use caution in cardiovascular disease.
Miscellaneous		
Bupropion (Wellbutrin, Wellbutrin SR)	100 mg bid; after at least 3 d, increase to 100 mg tid as needed [75, 100 mg] Sustained release: 100-200 mg bid [100, 150 mg]	Side effects: Agitation, dry mouth, insomnia, headache, nausea, constipation, tremor. Good choice for patients with sexual side effects from other agents; contraindicated in seizure disorders.
Maprotiline (Ludiomil)	75 to 225 in single or divided doses [25, 50, 75 mg].	Delays cardiac conduction; high anticholinergic activity; contraindicated in seizure disorders.
Mirtazepine (Remeron)	15 to 45 PO qd [15, 30 mg]	High anticholinergic activity; contraindicated in seizure disorders.
Nefazodone (Serzone)	Start at 100 mg PO bid, increase to 150-300 mg PO bid as needed [100, 150, 200, 250 mg].	Headache, somnolence, dry mouth, blurred vision. Postural hypotension, impotence.
Trazodone (Desyrel, generics)	150 mg/d, increasing by 50 mg/d every 3-4 d 400 mg/d in divided doses [50, 100, 150, 300 mg]	Rarely associated with priapism. Orthostatic hypotension in elderly. Sedating.
Venlafaxine (Effexor)	75 mg/d in 2-3 divided doses with food; increase to 225 mg/d as needed. [25, 37.5, 50, 75, 100 mg].	Inhibits norepinephrine and serotonin. Side effects: hypertension, nausea, somnolence, insomnia, dizziness, abnormal ejaculation, headache, dry mouth, anxiety.

IV. Mixed serotonin-norepinephrine inhibitors

A. Tricyclic antidepressants (TCAs) and SSRIs are equivalent in efficacy for the treatment of depression. Anticholinergic effects, weight gain, sedation, and orthostatic hypotension are most troubling with amitriptyline, clomipramine, doxepin, imipramine, and trimipramine. Amoxapine, desipramine, maprotiline, nortriptyline and protriptyline cause less sedation and fewer anticholinergic effects.

B. TCAs are toxic in overdose, and patients at risk for suicide must be given limited amounts to avoid the potential for suicide. A lethal TCA dose for an adult is only three to five times the therapeutic dose, or a 1-week supply of the antidepressant.

C. **Venlafaxine (Effexor)** is effective in treating severe, melancholic depression that has been unresponsive to other agents. Hypertension has been reported; therefore, this drug is usually reserved for patients unresponsive to first-line antidepressants.

D. Mixed serotonin effects

1. **Trazodone (Desyrel)** is very sedating, which can be beneficial for insomnia caused by depression. It is sometimes used along with an SSRI in patients who have difficulty sleeping. It has fewer anticholinergic side effects than many of the TCAs, but it can cause postural hypotension, and it has been associated with priapism.

2. **Nefazodone (Serzone)** is related to trazodone, but appears to have a more favorable side-effect profile. Sexual dysfunction has not been reported.

V. Mixed norepinephrine-dopamine reuptake inhibitors

A. Bupropion (Wellbutrin) has similar efficacy to that of the SSRIs and TCAs, and efficacy has been shown in patients previously unresponsive to TCAs. Side effects can include agitation and insomnia, psychosis, confusion, and weight loss. Bupropion is contraindicated in patients with seizure disorders.

VI. Adjunct therapy. Combined treatment may be beneficial in patients with incomplete response to a single antidepressant. A low-dose TCA or trazodone is often used along with an SSRI. Triiodothyronine may increase the efficacy of antidepressants.

References: See page 195.

Generalized Anxiety Disorder

Generalized anxiety disorder (GAD), is characterized by unrealistic or excessive anxiety and worry about two or more life circumstances for at least six months.

I. Clinical evaluation

A. Chronic worry is a prominent feature of GAD as opposed to the intermittent terror that characterizes panic disorder. Patients may report that they "can't stop worrying," which may revolve around life concerns relating to money, job, marriage, health, and safety of children.

B. Other features of GAD include insomnia, irritability, trembling, dry mouth, and a heightened startle reflex.

C. Symptoms of depression should be sought because 30-50% of patients with anxiety disorders will also have depression. Drugs and alcohol may contribute to anxiety disorders.

II. Medical disorders causing anxiety symptoms

A. Hyperthyroidism may cause anxiety, tachycardia, palpitations, sweating, dyspnea.

B. Cardiac rhythm disturbances and mitral valve prolapse may cause anxiety symptoms.

C. Substance abuse or dependence with withdrawal symptoms may resemble anxiety.

D. Pharmacologic causes of anxiety include salicylate intoxication, NSAIDs antihistamine intoxication/withdrawal, phenylpropanolamine pseudo-ephedrine, psychotropics (akathisia), stimulants, selective serotonin reuptake inhibitors. Caffeine, cocaine, amphetamines, theophylline, beta-agonists, over-the-counter decongestants, steroids, and marijuana can cause anxiety.

III. Laboratory evaluation of anxiety disorders

A. Chemistry profile (glucose, calcium, phosphate), TSH.

B. Special Tests. Urine drug screen, cortisol, serum catecholamine level.

IV. Treatment of Anxiety

A. Caffeinated beverages and excess alcohol should be avoided. Daily exercise and adequate sleep (with the use of medication if necessary) should be advised.

B. Buspirone (BuSpar)

1. Buspirone is a first line treatment of GAD. Buspirone requires 3-6 weeks at a dosage of 10-20 mg tid for efficacy. It lacks sedative effects. There is no physiologic dependence or withdrawal syndrome.
2. Combined benzodiazepine-buspirone therapy may be used for generalized anxiety disorder, with subsequent tapering of the benzodiazepine after 2-4 weeks.
3. Previous treatment with benzodiazepines or a history of substance abuse have a decreases the response to buspirone. Buspirone may have some antidepressant effects.

C. Antidepressants

1. Tricyclic antidepressants are widely used to treat anxiety disorders. Their onset of action is much slower than that of the benzodiazepines, but they have no addictive potential and may be more effective. An antidepressant is the agent of choice when depression is present in addition to anxiety.
2. Sedating antidepressants often have an early effect of promoting better sleep, although 2-3 weeks may pass before a patient experiences an antianxiety benefit. Better sleep usually brings some relief from symptoms, and the patient's functional level begins to improve almost immediately.
3. Anxious patients benefit from the sedating effects of imipramine (Tofranil), amitriptyline (Elavil), and doxepin (Sinequan). The daily dosage should be at least 50-100 mg.
4. Desipramine (Norpramin) is useful if sedation is not desired. The selective serotonin reuptake inhibitors (fluoxetine [Prozac]) may worsen anxiety symptoms before relieving them.

D. Benzodiazepines

1. Benzodiazepines can almost always relieve anxiety if given in adequate doses, and they have no delayed onset of action. Benzodiazepines should be reserved for patients who have failed to respond to buspirone and antidepressants or who are intolerant to their side effects.
2. Benzodiazepines are very useful for treating anxiety during the period in which it takes buspirone or antidepressants to exert their effects. Benzodiazepines should then be tapered after several weeks.
3. Benzodiazepines have few side effects other than sedation. Tolerance to their sedative effects develops, but not to their antianxiety properties.
4. Since clonazepam (Klonopin) and diazepam (Valium) have long half-lives, they are less likely to result in interdose anxiety and are easier to taper.
5. Drug dependency develops if the benzodiazepine is used regularly for more than 2-3 weeks. A withdrawal syndrome occurs in 70% of patients, including intense anxiety, tremulousness dysphoria, sleep and perceptual disturbances and appetite suppression. Slow tapering of benzodiazepines is crucial.
6. Patients with depression and anxiety should not receive benzodiazepines because they may worsen depression.
7. Benzodiazepines can be used in conjunction with an antidepressant. Therapy starts with alprazolam and an SSRI or tricyclic antidepressant. Alprazolam is then tapered after 2-3 weeks.

Anti-Anxiety Agent Dosages		
Drug	Dosage	Comments
Benzodiazepines		
Alprazolam (Xanax)	0.25-0.5 mg tid; increase by 1 mg/d at 3-4 day intervals to 0.75-4 mg/d [0.25, 0.5, 1, 2 mg]	Intermediate onset. Least sedating drug in class. Strong potential for dependence
Chlordiazepoxide (Librium, generics)	5 mg tid; 15-100 mg/d [5, 10, 25 mg]	Intermediate onset
Clonazepam (Klonopin)	0.5 mg tid; 1.5-20 mg/d [0.5, 1, 2 mg]	Intermediate onset. Long half-life; much less severe withdrawal
Clorazepate (Tranxene, generics)	7.5 mg bid; 15-60 mg/d [3.75, 7.5, 15 mg]	Fast onset
Diazepam (Valium, generics)	2 mg bid; 4-40 mg/d [2, 5, 10 mg]	Very fast onset
Halazepam (Paxipam)	20-40 mg tid-qid; 80-160 mg/d [20, 40 mg]	Intermediate to slow onset
Lorazepam (Ativan, generics)	1 mg bid; 2-6 mg/d [0.5, 1, 2 mg]	Intermediate onset
Oxazepam (Serax, generics)	10 mg tid; 30-120 mg/d [10, 15, 30 mg]	Intermediate to slow onset
Antidepressants		
Buspirone (BuSpar)	10 mg bid; max 60 mg/d; increase to 10 mg tid prn [5, 10, 15 mg dividose]	Antidepressant; nonaddicting, nonsedating. Not for prn usage; requires 2-3 wk to become effective.
Amitriptyline (Elavil, generics)	75 mg/d qhs-bid, increasing to 150-200 mg/d [25, 50, 75, 100, 150 mg]	Sedating, high anticholinergic activity
Doxepin (Sinequan, generics)	75 mg qhs or bid, max 300 mg/d [10, 25, 50, 75, 100, 150 mg]	A tricyclic antidepressant with antianxiety effects.

References: See page 195.

Panic Disorder

Panic disorder is an anxiety disorder characterized by unexpected panic attacks. It is often associated with situational avoidance stemming from fear of further attacks. Panic disorder has a lifetime prevalence between 1.5-3.0 percent, and it has a familial tendency.

I. Clinical diagnosis of panic disorder

A. Panic disorder is characterized by unexpected panic attacks. A panic attack is defined as a discrete episode of intense symptoms that peak within 10 minutes and primarily involve sympathetic nervous system manifestations.

B. A diagnosis of panic disorder is made if the patient has experienced recurrent, unexpected panic attacks and shows at least one of the following characteristics: (1) persistent concern about having another attack (anticipatory anxiety); (2) worry about the implications of an attack or its consequences (eg, suffering a catastrophic medical or mental consequence), or (3) a significant change in behavior related to the attacks.

C. **Agoraphobia** usually accompanies panic disorder. Agoraphobia refers to avoidance behavior motivated by fear of having another panic attack. It may consist of avoidance of activities that patients fear could provoke an attack, situations where escape may not be readily available, or activities during which patients are not accompanied by a person whom they believe could help in case of an attack.

Diagnostic Criteria for Panic Disorder, DSM-IV

A panic attack must include at least four of the following symptoms:

Neurologic symptoms
    Dizzy, light-headed or unsteady feeling
    Paresthesias
    Trembling/shaking
    Fainting
Cardiac symptoms
    Chest pain or discomfort
    Palpitations, heart pounding or tachycardia
    Sweating
Respiratory symptoms
    Shortness of breath
    Feeling of smothering or choking
Gastrointestinal symptoms
    Nausea
    Abdominal distress
Psychologic symptoms
    Derealization/depersonalization
    Fear of losing control, going crazy or dying
Miscellaneous symptoms
    Chills or hot flushes

Clinical Evaluation of Panic Symptoms

Assess characteristics of the panic attacks
Agoraphobic avoidance
Use of caffeine and other anxiety-provoking substances
Substance-use history
Medical history to eliminate organic etiology
Psychiatric comorbidity (eg, depression, interpersonal conflicts)
Previous assessments and treatments (psychiatric, medical)
Family history

II. Clinical management of panic disorder

A. **Tricyclic antidepressants**

1. Imipramine (Tofranil) and clomipramine (Anafranil) are considered first-line treatment options for panic disorder. The onset of therapeutic action

   for these tricyclic antidepressants typically takes three to four weeks.
2. Approximately one fourth of patients cannot tolerate the side effects of tricyclic antidepressants, which include constipation, dry mouth, blurred vision, urinary retention, sedation, weight gain, and orthostatic hypotension.
3. One of the most burdensome adverse effects for patients with panic disorder is the "activation syndrome," which occurs on initial titration in 25-40%. The syndrome often can be mitigated by initiating a low starting dosage (eg, 10 mg of imipramine per day), then increasing gradually at a rate of 10 mg every two to three days until a dosage of 50 to 75 mg is achieved. A withdrawal syndrome may occur following abrupt cessation of these agents.

Drugs Used For Treating Panic Disorder	
Drug	Dosage range
Tricyclic antidepressants Imipramine (Tofranil) Clomipramine (Anafranil) Nortriptyline (Pamelor) Desipramine (Norpramin)	50 to 300 mg per day 25 to 250 mg per day 25 to 100 mg per day 25 to 300 mg per day
SSRIs Fluoxetine (Prozac) Paroxetine (Paxil) Sertraline (Zoloft) Fluvoxamine (LuVox)	20 to 80 mg per day 10 to 50 mg per day 50 to 200 mg per day 50 to 300 mg per day
Benzodiazepines Alprazolam (Xanax) Lorazepam (Ativan) Clonazepam (Klonopin)	2 to 10 mg per day 2 to 6 mg per day 1 to 3 mg per day

B. Selective serotonin reuptake inhibitors
1. Fluvoxamine (LuVox) has been shown to be effective in placebo-controlled studies. Fluoxetine (Prozac), sertraline (Zoloft) and paroxetine (Paxil) may also be effective.
2. SSRIs are better tolerated than the tricyclics. Common side effects of SSRIs include sleep disturbance, headaches, gastrointestinal problems and sexual dysfunction. A withdrawal reaction may occur with abrupt cessation of SSRI therapy.
3. The SSRIs are appropriate first-line treatment for panic disorder, especially in patients with comorbid depression.
C. Benzodiazepines
1. Benzodiazepines are effective in the treatment of panic disorder. An advantage of the benzodiazepines is their quick onset of action relative to alternative agents, making them the only option for managing acutely distressed patients.
2. The principal drawback of benzodiazepines, particularly short-acting medications such as alprazolam (Xanax), is their ability to produce physical dependency, manifested by a withdrawal syndrome on abrupt discontinuation.
3. Benzodiazepines are considered an appropriate first-line treatment when rapid symptom relief is needed; however, discontinuation difficulties have relegated these medications to a second-line consideration. The most common use for benzodiazepines is to stabilize severe initial symptoms

until another treatment (e.g., an SSRI or cognitive behavioral therapy) becomes effective.

References: See page 195.

Insomnia

Insomnia affects about 35% of adults, and the incidence of sleep problems increases with age. Younger persons are apt to have trouble falling asleep, whereas older persons tend to have prolonged awakenings during the night.

I. **Causes of insomnia**
   A. **Situational stress** concerning job loss or problems, or an illness in the family often disrupt sleep. Patients under stress may experience interference with sleep onset and early morning awakening. Attempting to sleep in a new place, changes in time zones, or changing bedtimes due to shift work may interfere with sleep. Exercise or overstimulation late in the day may cause insomnia.
   B. **Drugs associated with insomnia** include antihypertensives, caffeine, diuretics, oral contraceptives, phenytoin, selective serotonin reuptake inhibitors, protriptyline, corticosteroids, stimulants, theophylline, and thyroid hormone.
   C. **Psychiatric disorders.** Depression is a common cause of poor sleep, often characterized by early morning awakening. Associated findings include hopelessness, sadness, loss of appetite, and reduced enjoyment of formerly pleasurable activities. Anxiety disorders and substance abuse may cause insomnia.
   D. **Medical disorders.** Prostatism, peptic ulcer, congestive heart failure, and chronic obstructive pulmonary disease may cause insomnia. Pain, nausea, dyspnea, cough, and gastroesophageal reflux may interfere with sleep.
   E. **Obstructive sleep apnea syndrome**
      1. This sleep disorder occurs in 5 to 15% of adults. It is characterized by recurrent discontinuation of breathing during sleep for at least 10 seconds. Abnormal oxygen saturation and sleep patterns result in excessive daytime fatigue and drowsiness. Loud snoring is typical. Overweight, middle-aged men are particularly predisposed to sleep apnea. Weight loss can be helpful in obese patients.
      2. Diagnosis is by polysomnography. Use of hypnotic agents is contraindicated since they increase the frequency and the severity of apneic episodes.

II. **Clinical evaluation of insomnia**
   A. Acute personal and medical problems should be sought, and the duration and pattern of symptoms and use of any psychoactive agents should be investigated. Substance abuse, leg movements, sleep apnea, loud snoring, nocturia, and daytime napping or fatigue should be sought.
   B. Consumption of caffeinated beverages, prescribed drugs, over-the-counter medications, and illegal substances should be sought.

III. **Behavioral therapy**
   A. A regular schedule of going to bed, arising, and eating meals should be recommended, and daytime naps discouraged. Daily exercise is helpful, but it should not be done in the late evening. Caffeine should not be consumed in the late afternoon or evening. Comfortable sleeping conditions should be assured, and the bed should be used only for sleeping and sexual activities.
   B. **Stimulus restriction.** Patients are advised to lie in bed only when they are sleepy and not when reading, eating, or watching television. If they do not fall asleep after a few minutes, they should get out of bed and read until they are sleepy. Use of ear plugs, a sleep mask, and a sound machine,

which reduces stimuli by emitting background noise, are often useful.
  C. **Sleep restriction** may be helpful. Each night, patients reduce the time in bed 30 minutes until reaching 4 hours per night; thereafter, they may add 15 minutes each night until 85% of time in bed is spent sleeping.
IV. **Pharmacologic therapy**
  A. **Zolpidem (Ambien)** is a nonbenzodiazepine imidazopyridine hypnotic agent which binds selectively to the benzodiazepine brain receptor. It is rapidly absorbed and has a short half-life and rapid onset of action. Zolpidem is not a drug of abuse potential, and it does not impair cognitive ability in the morning. The 10-mg tablet is prescribed for most patients, but elderly or medically ill patients should be given the 5-mg tablet. Rapid eye movement sleep is reduced without significant alterations of other sleep stages.
  B. **Triazolam (Halcion)** is a good initial choice in patients who have difficulty falling asleep because of a short half-life; it is quickly eliminated and causes no next-day sedation.
  C. **Temazepam (Restoril)** is useful in the elderly because excessive accumulation is less likely.
  D. **Effects of benzodiazepines on sleep.** Slow wave sleep and rapid eye movement (REM) sleep are reduced; REM sleep latency is prolonged. REM sleep and slow wave sleep have important functions in learning, memory, and adaptation to stress.
  E. **Sedating antidepressants,** such as trazodone (Desyrel) 150-400 mg qhs, doxepin (Sinequan) 25-150 mg qhs, or amitriptyline (Elavil) 25-75 mg qhs, can also be used to treat insomnia and are especially useful when the patient has underlying depression.

Sedative-Hypnotic Agents

Drug	Dosage	Half-life (hrs)	Side Effects	Positive Effects
Zolpidem (Ambien)	10 mg; 5 mg in elderly [5, 10 mg]	3-8	Potential for idio-syncratic side effects. Short acting.	Daytime alertness after use; lack of withdrawal; no suppression of REM.
Flurazepam (Dalmane)	15-30 mg [15, 30 mg]	48-120	Daytime drowsiness, confusion; sedative interactions. Intermediate- to long-acting.	Suppresses daytime anxiety; relative lack of withdrawal.
Triazolam (Halcion)	0.125-0.5 mg [0.125, 0.25 mg]	2-6	Amnesia; confusion; rebound insomnia; Abrupt onset and offset of action. Side effects can be unpredictable.	Short duration results in less daytime sedation.
Temazepam (Restoril)	15-30 mg [7.5, 15, 30 mg]	8-20	Rebound insomnia. Has slowest onset (30-60 min)	Daytime alertness after use. Short- to intermediate-acting.

Drug	Dosage	Half-life (hrs)	Side Effects	Positive Effects
Estazolam (ProSom)	1-2 mg [1, 2 mg]	8-24	REM sleep suppression; withdrawal symptoms. Daytime sedation	Short- to intermediate-acting.
Quazepam (Doral)	15 mg [7.5, 15 mg]	48-120	Daytime drowsiness, confusion; sedative interactions. Intermediate- to long-acting.	Lack of withdrawal effects; daytime alertness after use. Intermediate- to long-acting.

References: See page 195.

Smoking Cessation Therapy

Smoking causes approximately 430,000 smoking deaths each year, accounting for 19.5% of all deaths. Smoking cessation treatments should be offered to every patient who smokes.

I. **Behavioral counseling**, either group or individual, can raise the rate of abstinence to 20%-25%. The primary goals are to change the mental processes of smoking, reinforce the benefits of nonsmoking, and teach skills to help the smoker avoid high-risk situations. Patients are advised to put the money they save in a jar and buy themselves something they couldn't afford before they quit.

II. **Smoking cessation pharmacotherapy**

    A. The symptoms of withdrawal begin within a few hours and peak at 24-48 hours after quitting. Anxiety, hostility and anger are the most common symptoms, along with a craving for cigarettes, difficulty concentrating, restlessness, and insomnia. Symptoms usually last about 4 weeks.

Treatments for smoking cessation		
Drug	**Dosage**	**Comments**
Nicotine gum (Nicorette)	2- or 4-mg piece/30 min	Available OTC; poor compliance
Nicotine patch (Habitrol, Nicoderm CQ)	1 patch/d for 6-12 wk, then taper for 4 wk	Available OTC; local skin reactions
Nicotine nasal spray (Nicotrol NS)	1-2 doses/h for 6-8 wk	Rapid nicotine delivery; nasal irritation initially
Nicotine inhaler (Nicotrol Inhaler)	6-16 cartridges/d for 12 wk	Mimics smoking behavior; provides low doses of nicotine

Bupropion (Zyban)	150 mg/day for 3 d, then titrate to 300 mg	Treatment initiated 1 wk before quit day; contraindicated with seizures, anorexia, heavy alcohol use

- B. **Nicotine polacrilex (Nicorette)** is available OTC. The patient should use 1-2 pieces per hour. A 2-mg dose is recommended for those who smoke fewer than 25 cigarettes per day, and 4 mg for heavier smokers. It is used for 6 weeks, followed by 6 weeks of tapering. Nicotine gum improves smoking cessation rates by about 40%-60%. Drawbacks include poor compliance and unpleasant taste. The smoker should be instructed to bite down on the gum to release the nicotine and then place it between the teeth and buccal mucosa to be absorbed.
- C. **Transdermal nicotine (Habitrol, Nicoderm, Nicotrol)** doubles abstinence rates compared with placebo, The patch is available OTC and is easier to use than the gum. It provides a plateau level of nicotine at about half that of what a pack-a-day smoker would normally obtain. The higher dose should be used for 6-12 weeks followed by 4 weeks of tapering. A new patch is applied daily. Skin reactions occur in up to a third of patients. Applying 0.5% triamcinolone cream (Kenalog) reduces the irritation. The patch may be combined with the gum.
- D. **Nicotine nasal spray (Nicotrol NS)** is available by prescription and is a good choice for patients who have not been able to quit with the gum or patch or for heavy smokers. It delivers a high level of nicotine, similar to smoking. Nicotine nasal spray doubles the rates of sustained abstinence. The spray is used 6-8 weeks, at 1-2 doses per hour (one puff in each nostril). Tapering over about 6 weeks. Side effects include nasal and throat irritation, headache, and eye watering.
- E. **Nicotine inhaler (Nicotrol Inhaler)** delivers nicotine orally via inhalation from a plastic tube. It is available by prescription and has a success rate of 28%, similar to nicotine gum. The inhaler has the advantage of avoiding some of the adverse effects of nicotine gum, and its mode of delivery more closely resembles the act of smoking. Dosages range from 6-16 cartridges/day over 12 weeks. Side effects include cough and throat irritation.
- F. **Bupropion (Zyban)** is appropriate for patients who have been unsuccessful using nicotine replacement. Bupropion reduces withdrawal symptoms and can be used in conjunction with nicotine replacement therapy. Cessation rates are 12% to 23%, and the treatment is associated with reduced weight gain. Bupropion is contraindicated with a history of seizures, anorexia, heavy alcohol use, or head trauma.

References: See page 195.

Anorexia Nervosa

The prevalence of anorexia nervosa is 0.5-1%. The prevalence among males in this age range is about one-tenth that of females. The mortality rate in anorexia nervosa is 6%.
- I. **Pathophysiology**
  - A. This disorder is characterized by: 1) a body weight that is below normal (ie, <85% of expected body weight); 2) intense fears of weight gain despite being underweight; 3) body image disturbance resulting in the misperception of one's weight or shape, undue self-evaluation based upon weight, or denial of the seriousness of the current low weight; and 4) in postmenarchal females, the absence of at least three consecutive menstrual cycles. The diagnosis of anorexia nervosa requires all four criteria.

    B. Restricting type anorexia nervosa is characterized by restrictive eating patterns. Binge-eating/purging type anorexia nervosa is characterized by binge-eating episodes followed by purging behavior.

    C. **A binge** consists of rapid intake of 2500 calories or 2.5 times the normal amount of food. Binges are characterized by a lack of control over food intake during a period of less than 2 hours.

    D. **Purging** behaviors entail acute and active efforts to eradicate ingested calories and may include self-induced vomiting and/or the use of laxatives, diuretics, or enemas.

II. Clinical evaluation of anorexia nervosa

    A. **Dieting behavior.** Indications of dieting behavior include preoccupation with body weight or specific body areas, attempts to restrict calories and fatty foods, frequent weighings, mirror gazing, preoccupation with food, meal avoidance, preoccupation with clothes size, and attempts to hide weight loss with bulky clothing.

    B. **Physical examination** should include blood pressure, height, and weight. Emaciation and evidence of slowed metabolic and physiological functions may be apparent. Lanugo, a fine, downy body hair, may be prominent on the arms, torso, and face.

    C. **Cardiovascular complications** are the most likely cause of death in anorexia nervosa. Bradycardia, orthostatic hypotension, and mitral valve prolapse are common.

    D. **Psychological assessment.** The patient may appear indifferent to the weight loss (denial), and mental status examination often reveals a flat affect and poor eye contact. The eyes may have a lackluster appearance due to the effects of starvation. Impairment of concentration, lack of cooperation, limited verbalization, and dysphoric mood are frequent.

    E. **A general laboratory screen** is usually sufficient in the assessment of anorexia nervosa. Among individuals who purge, determination of electrolyte status is the most important concern, particularly serum potassium status. An electrocardiogram is indicated for cardiac symptoms, extremely low body weight, or history of exposure to syrup of ipecac.

Laboratory Abnormalities in Anorexia Nervosa

Anemia	Hypokalemia (vomiting, laxatives, diuretics)
Leukopenia	Hypercortisolemia
Thrombocytopenia	Hypoglycemia
Reduced erythrocyte sedimentation rate	Elevated growth hormone levels
Impaired cell-mediated immunity	Reduced estrogen levels
Hypercholesterolemia	Reduced basal levels of luteinizing and follicle-stimulating hormones
Hypocalcemia	Elevated liver function tests
Hypomagnesemia	Elevated amylase (vomiting)
Hypophosphatemia	

III. Management of anorexia nervosa

    A. The patient should be weighed at each visit. In individuals not previously overweight, weight loss of more than 25% of the previous body weight requires referral to a structured refeeding program in an inpatient or day treatment program. Outpatient psychological management is indicated for lesser degrees of weight loss. In amenorrheic patients, bone mass should be protected with hormonal replacement therapy. Psychological intervention may include a structured outpatient refeeding program, cognitive-behavioral therapy, individual psychotherapy, and/or group or family therapy. Support groups may also be helpful.

    B. Suicidal ideation requires psychiatric hospitalization, and depression

requires antidepressant treatment. Anti-depressants with anti-obsessional features (ie, selective serotonin reuptake inhibitors) are recommended.
  C. Fluoxetine (Prozac) has been used successfully in the therapy of anorexia and bulimia; 20 mg PO qAM.
  D. For patients who induce vomiting, fluoride treatments may improve dentition. Laxative-dependent patients should be gradually weaned off laxatives, and dietary fiber should be gradually increased and adequate hydration maintained.
IV. **Prognosis**. About one-third of patients fully recover, one-third improve, and one-third remain impaired. This latter third frequently also have personality disorders or depression.

References: See page 195.

Bulimia Nervosa

Bulimia nervosa is characterized by binge eating and inappropriate vomiting, fasting, excessive exercise and the misuse of diuretics, laxatives or enemas. Bulimia nervosa is 10 times more common in females than in males and affects up to 3 percent of young women. The condition usually becomes symptomatic between the ages of 13 and 20 years.

Diagnostic Criteria for Bulimia Nervosa, DSM IV

A. **Recurrent episodes of binge eating.** An episode of binge eating is characterized by both of the following:
  1. Eating, in a discrete period of time (e.g., within a two-hour period), an amount of food that is definitely larger than most people would eat during a similar period of time and under similar circumstances.
  2. A sense of lack of control over eating during the episode (e.g., a feeling that one cannot stop eating or control what or how much one is eating).
B. Recurrent inappropriate compensatory behavior in order to prevent weight gain, such as self-induced vomiting; misuse of laxatives, diuretics, enemas, or other medications; fasting or excessive exercise.
C. The binge eating and inappropriate compensatory behaviors both occur, on average, at least twice a week for three months.
D. Self-evaluation is unduly influenced by body shape and weight.
E. The disturbance does not occur exclusively during episodes of anorexia nervosa.
Specify type:
  Purging type: during the current episode of bulimia nervosa, the person has regularly engaged in self-induced vomiting or the misuse of laxatives, diuretics, or enemas.
  Nonpurging type: during the current episode of bulimia nervosa, the person has used other inappropriate compensatory behaviors, such as fasting or excessive exercise, but has not regularly engaged in self-induced vomiting or the misuse of laxatives, diuretics, or enemas.

I. **Pathophysiology of bulimia nervosa**
  A. Bulimia nervosa may have a genetic predisposition. Other predisposing factors include psychologic and personality factors, such as perfectionism, impaired self-concept, affective instability, poor impulse control and an

absence of adaptive functioning to maturational tasks and developmental stressors (eg, puberty, peer and parental relationships, sexuality, marriage and pregnancy).
B. Bulimia nervosa appears to have a chronic, sometimes episodic course in which periods of remission alternate with recurrences of binge/purge cycles. Thirty percent of patients with bulimia nervosa rapidly relapse and up to 40 percent remain chronically symptomatic.
C. Comorbid major depression is commonly noted. There is an increased incidence of rapid cycling mood disorders and anxiety and substance-related disorders. Substance abuse involving alcohol and stimulants, occurs in one third of patients with bulimia nervosa. Between 2 and 50 percent of women with bulimia nervosa have borderline, antisocial, histrionic or narcissistic personality disorder.

II. Medical complications
A. Medical complications of bulimia nervosa include fatigue, bloating and constipation, to chronic or life-threatening conditions, including hypokalemia, cathartic colon, impaired renal function and cardiac arrest.
B. **Binge eating** may cause gastric rupture, the most serious complication, is uncommon. More often, patients describe nausea, abdominal pain and distention, prolonged digestion and weight gain. The combination of heightened anxiety, physical discomfort and intense guilt provokes the drive to purge the food by self-induced vomiting, excessive exercise or the misuse of ipecac, laxatives or diuretics. These purgative methods are associated with the more serious complications of bulimia nervosa.
C. **Self-induced vomiting** is used by more than 75 percent of patients with bulimia nervosa. Most patients vomit immediately or soon after a binge. Vomiting is induced by stimulation of the pharynx using a finger or a narrow object such as a toothbrush. Self-induced vomiting can lead to a number of serious medical complications, such as depletions of chloride, potassium, sodium and magnesium. Hypokalemia is a potential medical emergency.

Medical Complications of Bulimia Nervosa

Type of Behavior	Complications
Binge eating	Gastric rupture, nausea, abdominal pain and distention, prolonged digestion
Purging (self-induced vomiting)	Dental erosion, enlarged salivary glands Oral/hand trauma, esophagitis, pharyngitis, upper gastrointestinal tears, hematemesis abdominal pain, hypokalemia, fatigue, muscle spasms, palpitations, paresthesias, tetany, seizures, arrhythmias

III. Patient evaluation
A. Psychiatric assessment
1. Evaluation should include general personality features, characterologic disturbance and attitudes about eating, body size and weight.
2. A complete history of the patient's body weight, eating patterns and attempts at weight loss, including typical daily food intake, methods of purging and perceived ideal weight should be obtained.
3. An investigation of the patient's interpersonal history and functioning, including family dynamics, peer relationships, and present or past physical, sexual or emotional abuse should be completed.
4. An evaluation of medical and psychiatric comorbidity, as well as documentation of previous attempts at treatment should be documented.

    B. Physical evaluation should include vital signs and an evaluation of height and weight relative to age. The physician should also look for general hair loss, lanugo, abdominal tenderness, acrocyanosis (cyanosis of the extremities), jaundice, edema, parotid gland tenderness or enlargement, and scars on the dorsum of the hand should be sought.

    C. Laboratory tests in patients with bulimia nervosa include a complete blood count with differential, serum chemistry and thyroid profiles, and urine chemistry microscopy testing. A chest radiograph and electrocardiogram may be indicated in some cases.

IV. Treatment

    A. Tricyclic antidepressants. Tricyclic antidepressants reduce binge eating by 47 to 91 percent and vomiting by 45 to 78 percent. Desipramine (Norpramin) , 150 to 300 mg per day, imipramine, 176 to 300 mg per day, and amitriptyline (Elavil), 150 mg per day, are recommended.

    B. Selective serotonin reuptake inhibitors. At the 20-mg dosage, fluoxetine (Prozac) therapy results in a 45 percent reduction in binge eating, compared with a 33 percent reduction with placebo. Vomiting was reduced by 29 percent. Fluoxetine in a dosage of 60 mg per day results in a 67 percent reduction in binge eating and a 56 percent reduction in vomiting.

    C. Psychotherapy

        1. Cognitive-behavioral therapy principally involves a systematic series of interventions aimed at addressing the cognitive aspects of bulimia nervosa, such as the preoccupation with body, weight and food, perfectionism, dichotomous thinking and low self-esteem. Therapy should address the behavioral components of the illness, such as disturbed eating habits, binge eating, purging, dieting and ritualistic exercise.

        2. The initial goal of cognitive-behavioral therapy is to restore control over dietary intake. Caloric restriction and dieting efforts should be discontinued. Patients should record their food intake and feelings and receive extensive feedback concerning their meal plan, symptom triggers, caloric intake and nutritional balance. Patients are instructed in methods for challenging rigid thought patterns, improving self-esteem, assertiveness training, and appropriate expression of feelings.

References: See page 195.

Drug and Alcohol Dependence

Nearly one half of all primary care patients have an alcohol or drug disorder. Each stage of addictive illness can be characterized by types and severity of withdrawal and relapse prevention.

I. Pharmacotherapy for withdrawal syndromes

    A. Detoxification. Pharmacologic therapies are indicated for use in patients with addictive disorders to prevent life-threatening withdrawal complications such as seizures and delirium tremens.

    B. Alcohol withdrawal. Agents that are commonly recommended include diazepam (Valium), lorazepam (Ativan), chlordiazepoxide (Limbitrol) and clorazepate (Tranxene). Longer-acting preparations such as diazepam or chlordiazepoxide provide a smoother and safer withdrawal than other preparations.

Signs and Symptoms of Alcohol and Drug Withdrawal

Drug	Peak period	Duration	Signs	Symptoms
Alcohol	1 to 3 days	5 to 7 days	Elevated blood pressure, pulse and temperature, hyperarousal, agitation, restlessness, cutaneous flushing, tremors, diaphoresis, dilated pupils, ataxia, clouding of consciousness, disorientation	Anxiety, panic, paranoid delusions, illusions, visual and auditory hallucinations
Benzodiazepines and other sedative/hypnotics	Short-acting: 2 to 4 days Long-acting: 4 to 7 days	Short-acting: 4 to 7 days Long-acting: 7 to 14 days	Increased psychomotor activity, agitation, muscular weakness, tremulousness, hyperpyrexia, diaphoresis, delirium, convulsions, elevated blood pressure, pulse and temperature, tremor	Anxiety, depression, euphoria, incoherent thoughts, hostility, grandiosity, disorientation, tactile, auditory and visual hallucinations, suicidal thoughts
Stimulants (cocaine, amphetamines and derivatives)	1 to 3 days	5 to 7 days	Social withdrawal, psychomotor retardation, hypersomnia, hyperphagia	Depression, anhedonia, suicidal thoughts and behavior, paranoid delusions
Opiates (heroin)	1 to 3 days	5 to 7 days	Drug seeking, mydriasis, piloerection, diaphoresis, rhinorrhea, lacrimation, diarrhea, insomnia, elevated blood pressure and pulse	Intense desire for drugs, muscle cramps, arthralgia, anxiety, nausea, vomiting, malaise
PCP/psychedelics	Days to weeks	Days to weeks	Hyperactivity, increased pain threshold, nystagmus, hyperreflexia, hypertension and tachycardia, eyelid retraction (stare), agitation and hyperarousal, dry and erythematous skin, violent and self-destructive behaviors	Anxiety, depression, delusions, auditory and visual hallucinations, memory loss, irritable and angry mood and affect, suicidal thoughts

Medications for Alcohol Detoxification

Mild withdrawal	Moderate withdrawal	Severe withdrawal (delirium tremens)	Loading-dose method
Diazepam (Valium),5 to 10 mg PO as needed.	Diazepam: 15 to 20 mg PO four times daily on day 1 10 to 20 mg PO four times daily on day 2. 5 to 15 mg PO four times daily on day 3 10 mg PO four times daily on day 4. 5 mg PO four times daily on day 5.	Diazepam, 10 to 25 mg PO as needed every hour while awake until sedation occurs.	Diazepam, 10 mg, or chlordiazepoxide (Limbitrol), 25 mg, PO every hour Diazepam may be given intravenously

Thiamine, 100 mg intramuscularly or PO every day for 3 to 7 days, hydration and magnesium replacement may be indicated, according to the severity of the withdrawal state.

II. **Benzodiazepines and other sedative/hypnotics.** The signs and symptoms of benzodiazepine withdrawal are similar to those for withdrawal from barbiturates. Withdrawal is not usually marked by significant elevations in blood pressure and pulse.

Benzodiazepine and Barbiturate Withdrawal

Short-acting detoxification	Long-acting detoxification
7- to 10-day taper: On day 1, give diazepam (Valium), 10 to 20 mg PO qid, and taper until the dosage is 5 to 10 mg PO on last day.	10- to 14-day taper: On day 1, give diazepam, 10 to 20 mg PO qid, and taper until the dosage is 5 to 10 mg PO on last day.

III. **Stimulants (cocaine, amphetamines and derivatives)**
   A. Supportive treatment is indicated in patients who are undergoing withdrawal from stimulants. Since stimulant withdrawal may cause significant irritability, a dosage of 5 to 10 mg of diazepam given PO q6h on a fixed schedule or as needed for two to three days is recommended in patients with mild to moderate withdrawal symptoms.
   B. For severe withdrawal symptoms with persistent depression, therapy may be initiated with desipramine (Norpramin), at a dosage of 50 mg per day, titrated upward every other day in 50-mg increments until a dosage of 150 to 250 mg per day is attained.
IV. **Opiates**. Management of withdrawal can be accomplished with clonidine (Catapres) or methadone. Federal regulations do not allow the use of methadone for detoxification if opiate withdrawal is the primary diagnosis.
V. **Phencyclidine and other psychedelic agents**. Acute symptoms of withdrawal from psychedelic agents may be diminished or reversed by using haloperidol (Haldol), 5 to 10 mg IM or PO every 3-6h prn. Lorazepam, 1 to 2 mg intravenously, or diazepam, 5 to 10 mg q3-6h prn, can also be given as needed.

VI. Medications for relapse prevention

A. Disulfiram (Antabuse)

1. Disulfiram is an aversive agent. The dosage of is 250 mg per day. Disulfiram inhibits acetaldehyde dehydrogenase. An accumulation of acetaldehyde produces an unpleasant reaction when alcohol is consumed that is similar to a severe hangover. It is potentially lethal, although only a small number of fatalities have been reported. The reaction is characterized by headache, diaphoresis, tachycardia, nausea and vomiting, cardiovascular collapse, delirium, seizures and, occasionally, death.

2. Before using disulfiram, patients must have a blood alcohol level of zero and must be able to comprehend the risks and benefits of treatment.

B. Methadone maintenance is a form of pharmacologic management of opiate addiction performed in programs that are in compliance with federal regulations.

C. Naltrexone (ReVia) is an opioid antagonist which inhibits the effect of opiate agonists. Naltrexone is effective in decreasing relapse and the subjective craving for alcohol.

References

References may be obtained via the internet at www.ccspublishing.com.

Index

Internet Journals from
Current Clinical Strategies Publishing

Journal of Primary Care Medicine
Journal of Medicine
Journal of Pediatrics and Adolescent Medicine
Journal of Surgery
Journal of Family Medicine
Journal of Emergency Medicine and Acute Primary
Care
Journal of Psychiatry
Journal of AIDS/HIV

www.ccspublishing.com